AF818284

Digestive Diseases

Current Concepts in Research and Practice

Formerly 'Survey of Digestive Diseases'

Editors-in-Chief

T.S.N. Chen, East Orange, N.J.
R.P. MacDermott, Philadelphia, Pa.

Editorial Board

Infectious Disease
E.C. Boedeker, Washington, D.C.

Radiology
P.S. Chen, Worcester, Mass.

Endoscopy
D. Fleischer, Washington, D.C.

Liver
P. Ferenci, Wien
T. Kiernan, Augusta, Ga.
K. Okuda, Chiba

Pharmacology
R.G. Knodell, Baltimore, Md.
C. Scarpignato, Parma

Bile
U.A. Marbet, Basel

Immunology
S. Kakumu, Nagoya

Esophagus and Stomach
S.K. Lam, Hong Kong
D.A. Peura, Washington, D.C.
R.K.H. Wong, Washington, D.C.

Colon
P. Rozen, Tel-Aviv

Preventive Medicine
C.H. Tamburro, Louisville, Ky.

Oncology
M. Tempero, Omaha, Nebr.

Pediatric Gastroenterology
J.A. Vanderhoof, Omaha, Nebr.

Surgery
L.F. Rikkers, Omaha, Nebr.
J.S. Thompson, Omaha, Nebr.

KARGER

Printed in Switzerland
on acid-free paper by
Thür AG Offsetdruck, Pratteln

Appears bimonthly:
1 volume per year (6 issues)

Digestive Diseases

Submission: Manuscripts should be addressed to:

Thomas S. Chen, MD
Department of Pathology (113)
VA Medical Center
East Orange, NJ 07019 (USA)
or
Richard P. MacDermott, MD
University of Pennsylvania
Gastroenterology Division
Suite 600/CRB
422 Curie Boulevard
Philadelphia, PA 19104–6144 (USA)

Manuscripts should be submitted in triplicate (with three sets of illustrations of which one is an original), typewritten double-spaced on one side of the paper, with a wide margin.

Conditions: Manuscripts must be written in English, and are all subject to editorial review. Manuscripts are received with the explicit understanding that they are not submitted for simultaneous consideration by any other publication. Submission of an article for publication implies the transfer of the copyright from the author to the publisher upon acceptance. Accepted papers become the permanent property of 'Digestive Diseases' and may not be reproduced by any means, in whole or in part, without the written consent of the publisher. It is the author's responsibility to obtain permission to reproduce illustrations, tables, etc. from other publications.

Arrangement

Title page: The first page of each paper should indicate the title (main title underlined), the authors' names, and the institute where the work was conducted. A short title for use as running head as well as the full address of the author to whom correspondence should be sent are also required.

Full address: The exact postal address complete with postalcode must be given at the bottom of the title page. Please also supply phone and fax numbers.

Key words: For indexing purposes, a list of 3–10 key words in English is essential.

Abstract: Each paper needs an abstract of up to 10 lines.

Small type: Paragraphs which can or must be set in smaller type (case histories, test methods, etc.) should be indicated with a 'p' (petit) in the margin on the left-hand side.

Footnotes: Avoid footnotes. When essential, they are numbered consecutively and typed at the foot of the appropriate page.

Tables and illustrations: Tables and illustrations (both numbered in Arabic numerals) should be prepared on separate sheets. Tables require a heading and figures a legend, also prepared on a separate sheet. For the reproduction of illustrations, only good drawings and original photographs can be accepted; negatives or photocopies cannot be used. When possible, group several illustrations on one block for reproduction (max. size 144 × 196 mm) or provide crop marks. On the back of each illustration, indicate its number, the author's name, and 'top'. Color illustrations are reproduced at the author's expense.

References: In the text identify references by Arabic numerals [in square brackets]. Material submitted for publication but not yet accepted should be noted as 'unpublished data' and not be included in the reference list. The list of references should include only those publications which are cited in the text. Do not alphabetize; number references in the order in which they are first mentioned in the text. The surnames of the authors followed by initials should be given. There should be no punctuation other than a comma to separate the authors. Cite all authors, 'et al' is not sufficient. Abbreviate journal names according to the Index Medicus system. (Also see International Committee of Medical Journal Editors: Uniform requirements for manuscripts submitted to biomedical journals. Br Med J 1988;296:401–405).

Examples

(a) Papers published in periodicals: Kauffman HF, van der Heide S, Beaumont F, Blok H, de Vries K: Class-specific antibody determination against *Aspergillus fumigatus* by means of the enzyme-linked immunosorbent assay. III. Comparative study: IgG, IgA, IgM ELISA titers, precipitating antibodies and IgE binding after fractionation of the antigen. Int Arch Allergy Appl Immunol 1986;80:300–306.

(b) Monographs: Matthews DE, Farewell VT: Using and Understanding Medical Statistics. Basel, Karger, 1985.

(c) Edited books: Hardy WD Jr, Essex M: FeLV-induced feline acquired immune deficiency syndrome: A model for human AIDS; in Klein E (ed): Acquired Immunodeficiency Syndrome. Prog Allergy. Basel, Karger, 1986, vol 37, pp 353–376.

Further details: Authors may consult our leaflet 'Rules for the Preparation of Manuscripts', available on request from the Publisher, S. Karger AG, P.O. Box, CH-4009 Basel (Switzerland).

Page charges: There is no page charge for papers of 8 or fewer printed pages (including tables, illustrations and references). Each additional complete or partial page is charged to the author at SFr. 225.– / US $ 150.00. The allotted size of a paper is equal to approx. 18 manuscript pages (including tables, illustrations and references).

Galley proofs: Unless indicated otherwise, galley proofs are sent to the first-named author and should be returned with the least possible delay. Alterations made in galley proofs, other than the correction of printer's errors, are charged to the author. No page proofs are supplied.

Reprints: Order forms and a price list are sent with the galley proofs. Orders submitted after the issue is printed are subject to considerably higher prices. Allow five weeks from date of publication for delivery of reprints.

KARGER

General Information

Digestive Diseases

Publication data: 'Digestive Diseases' is published 6 times annually. Volume 10 with 6 issues appears in 1992.
Subscription rates: Subscriptions run for a full calendar year. Prices are given per volume, surface postage included.
Personal subscription:
SFr. 226.50, US$ 151.00.
(Must be in the name of, billed to, and paid by an individual. Order must be marked 'personal subscription'.)
Institutional subscription:
(Regular rate.) SFr. 453.–, US$ 302.00.
Residents: SFr. 158.55, US$ 105.70.
Airmail postage: SFr. 35.–, US$ 30.00.
(Extra per volume.)
Microform subscription:
SFr. 226.50, US$ 151.00.
(Available exclusively to subscribers of the paper edition.)
Single issues and back volumes: Information on availability and prices can be obtained through the Publisher.
Advertising: Correspondence and rate requests should be addressed to the Publisher.

Subscription orders: Orders can be placed at agencies, bookstores, directly with the Publisher S. Karger AG, P.O. Box, CH – 4009 Basel (Switzerland) or with any of the following distributors:
Deutschland:
S. Karger GmbH, Lörracher Strasse 16A
Postfach, D-W-7800 Freiburg
France: Librairie Luginbühl
36, bd de Latour-Maubourg
F–75007 Paris
Great Britain, Ireland:
S. Karger Publishers,
11 Ravenscroft Road
Beckenham, Kent BR3 4TP
USA: S. Karger Publishers, Inc.
26 West Avon Road, P.O. Box 529
Farmington, CT 06085
India, Bangladesh, Sri Lanka:
S. Karger India Subscription Agency
B – 5/132 Safdarjung Enclave
New Delhi-110029
Japan: Katakura Libri, Inc.
36-9 Hongo 3-chome, Bunkyo-ku
Tokyo 113
Change of address: Both old and new address should be stated and sent to the subscription source.

Bibliographic indices: This journal is regularly listed in bibliographic services, including *Current Contents®*.
Book Reviews: Books are accepted for review by special agreement.
Copying: This journal has been registered with the Copyright Clearance Center (CCC), as indicated by the code appearing on the first page of each article. For readers in the US, this code signals consent for copying of articles for personal or internal use, or for the personal or internal use of specific clients, provided that the stated fee is paid per copy directly to CCC, 21 Congress Street, Salem, MA 01970 (USA). A copy of the first page of the article must accompany payment. Consent does not extend to copying for general distribution, for promotion, for creating new works, or for resale. In these cases, specific written permission must be obtained from the copyright owner, S. Karger AG, P.O. Box, CH – 4009 Basel (Switzerland).

KARGER

Gastroenterology in Karger Journals

Chirurgische Gastroenterologie

DIGESTION

Digestive Diseases

Digestive Surgery

S. Karger Publishers produce over 80 medical and scientific journals covering a wide range of specialties. Several of these are of specific interest to gastroenterologists.

Full details may be found in the Karger Journals Catalogue.

KARGER

Please ask for free sample copies

KI 93021

World Review of Nutrition and Dietetics
(ISSN 0084–2230), **Vol. 68**
Series Editor: A.P. Simopoulos, Washington, D.C.

Editors: Artemis P. Simopoulos, Ritva R. Butrum

International Food Data Bases and Information Exchange

Concepts, Principles
and Designs

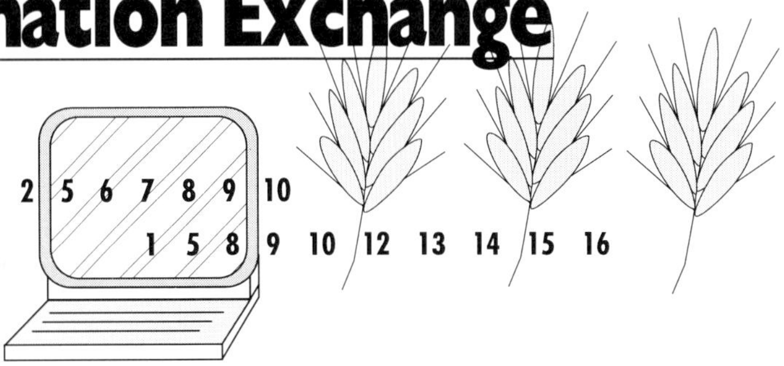

Information on the nutritive and nonnutritive components of foods is essential for our understanding of the role of nutrition in human health. The quality, quantity and accessibility of these data constitute an important resource for health professionals concerned with the food supply and its implications for the overall health of individuals and population groups throughout the world. This volume brings together the most up-to-date information on international food data bases and the issues involved in their development. Experts at the forefront of research describe not only the strengths and weaknesses of the various systems in place but also current initiatives to standardize and document procedures for maintaining timely and reliable data bases. Special attention is also given to principles for the preparation of food composition tables, the need for an international food description language and plans for the design and implementation of a single International Food Data Base.

As the first publication to describe and evaluate existing models and systems on food composition, this book is essential reading for everyone working in human nutrition as well as for policy makers, consumers and those involved in food marketing.

Contents

Fields of Interest

Nutrition; Biochemistry, Dietetics, Epidemiology, General Medicine, Public Health

World Review of Nutrition and Dietetics, Vol. 68
International Food Data Bases and Information Exchange
Concepts, Principles and Designs
Editors: Simopoulos, A.P. (Washington, D.C.); Butrum, R.R. (Rockville, Md.)
XII + 160 p., 22 fig., 21 tab., hard cover, 1992
SFr. 186.– / DM 223.– / £ 93.00 / US$ 149.00
Prices subject to change
DM price for FRG, £ price for UK, US$ price for USA only
ISBN 3–8055–5480–X

KARGER

KI 92532

Controversies about Inflammatory Diseases of the Pancreas

Guest Editors
C. Beglinger, Basel
U. Marbet, Altdorf

5 figures, 1 color plate, 12 tables, 1992

KARGER

S. Karger
Medical and Scientific Publishers
Basel · Freiburg · Paris · London
New York · New Delhi · Bangkok
Singapore · Tokyo · Sydney

Drug Dosage
The authors and the publisher have exerted every effort to ensure that drug selection and dosage set forth in this text are in accord with current recommendations and practice at the time of publication. However, in view of ongoing research, changes in government regulations, and the constant flow of information relating to drug therapy and drug reactions, the reader is urged to check the package insert for each drug for any change in indications and dosage and for added warnings and precautions. This is particularly important when the recommended agent is a new and/or infrequently employed drug.

All rights reserved.
No part of this publication may be translated into other languages, reproduced or utilized in any form or by any means, electronic or mechanical, including photocopying, recording, microcopying, or by any information storage and retrieval system, without permission in writing from the publisher or, in the case of photocopying, direct payment of a specified fee to the Copyright Clearance Center (see 'Information for Readers and Subscribers').

© Copyright 1992 by S. Karger AG,
P.O. Box, CH-4009 Basel (Switzerland)
Printed in Switzerland on acid-free paper by
Thür AG Offsetdruck, Pratteln
ISBN 3-8055-5719-1

Contents

Dig Dis 1992;10:317

Ch. Beglinger, Basel
U.A. Marbet, Altdorf

Foreword

Over the past years our knowledge on the physiology, pathobiology and treatment of pancreatic diseases has increased substantially. Despite this progress, many aspects remain controversial and treatment modalities are still a matter of debate. In this overview we would like to focus on different practical problems with which every physician, who is dealing with pancreatic diseases, is confronted daily.

The risk factors for developing chronic pancreatitis and the natural history has been reviewed by R. Münch. Alcohol remains not only the main risk factor, at least in developed western countries, but is also the most frequent cause of persistent chronic pain which remains a challenge for every clinician and surgeon, as discussed by H.G. Gooszen. Patients should not be withheld from the surgeon, until the chronic pancreatitis has burned out and been replaced by problems of pancreatic insufficiency. The basic aspects of physiology in chronic pancreatitis are discussed by Ch. Beglinger.

Prognostic uncertainty upon admission of patients with acute pancreatitis hampers correct treatment. In the past years computer tomography has proven to be of great help to recognize patients at risk for developing life-threatening complications and to follow patients during acute disease, a topic adressed by P. Meyer and coworkers. In addition, endoscopic retrograde cholangiography with papillotomy may be neccessary if a common bile duct stone is suspected and the course of the disease does not improve spontaneously during the first 48 h. Although this approach is still a matter of debate, different theoretical and clinical evaluations support the strategy as concluded by U. Marbet. The role of surgery in pancreatic disease has been critically discussed by M. Büchler and co-workers. The surgical removal of contaminated necrotic material in patients with local septic complications following acute pancreatitis is widely accepted. In single patients with fulminant disease, even surgical intervention during the first 3–5 days may be of benefit.

We hope that these practically oriented reviews contribute to a better understanding and management of pancreatic diseases.

Dig Dis 1992;10:318–325

U.A. Marbet

Department of Medicine,
Kantonsspital Uri, Altdorf,
Switzerland

Gallstone-Associated Acute Pancreatitis: A Field for Endoscopic Therapy?

Key Words

Gallstone-associated pancreatitis
Common bile duct stone
Endoscopic treatment of pancreatitis

Abstract

The pathogenesis of acute pancreatitis even if associated with gallstone remains unclear. This explains that the best treatment for gallstone-associated pancreatitis remains a matter of debate. However, different theoretical and clinical evaluations support the strategy to perform an endoscopic papillotomy if a common bile duct stone is suspected and the course of the disease does not improve spontaneously during the first 48 h. The discrepancies of the current data and the difficulties to give rational suggestions have been reviewed.

The best treatment for gallstone-associated acute pancreatitis is still evolving. Most of the stones in the common bile duct responsible for acute pancreatitis pass spontaneously and up to 80% of the patients resolve without specific treatment. In addition, the pathogenesis of severe pancreatitis is far from clear and we have no definite possibility to predict the outcome of the biliary obstruction and the course of the disease with accuracy early in the disease explaining the persisting controversy on the optimal treatment. In this review we would like to focus on the discrepancies of the current data and the difficulties to give rational suggestions on how best to treat gallstone-associated acute pancreatitis.

Etiology and Pathogenesis of Acute Pancreatitis

Etiologies of acute pancreatitis include a long list of sometimes unproven conditions associated with acute pancreatitis (table 1) [1] up to organic solvents like polychlorinated biphenyls [2] and antibiotics like metronida-

U. Marbet, MD
Department of Medicine
Kantonsspital Uri
CH–6460 Altdorf (Switzerland)

© 1992
S. Karger AG, Basel
0257–2753/92/
0106–0318$2.75/0

zole [3], which have also recently been considered as responsible causes of acute pancreatitis. Excess of alcohol and biliary tract disease, however, still represent at least 80% of the cases.

In a study from Milwaukee [4], 116 patients with idiopathic recurrent pancreatitis have been studied by endoscopic retrograde cholangiopancreaticography (ERCP). Thirty-eight percent of patients were deemed to have a surgically or endoscopically remediable condition, gallstone being one of them. This study not only supports the need for endoscopic evaluation in patients with pancreatitis of unknown etiology, but also emphasizes biliary changes as an important cause of acute pancreatitis.

However, the pathogenesis of acute pancreatitis, even if associated with gallstone, still remains unclear. Autodigestion has been considered for many years as the main pathogenetic principle in acute pancreatitis [1]. Different observations support this hypothesis. Trypsin seems to be activated in acute pancreatitis as suggested by the fall of 2-macroglobulin, the principal inhibitor of serine proteases in plasma, and the abnormal high proportion of circulating 2-macroglobulin in the form of complexes with enzymes [5]. In addition, trypsinogen activation peptides have been demonstrated in the urine [6] of patients with acute pancreatitis. Changes in blood flow, increased membrane permeability, alteration of cellular metabolism, free radicals, suspected imbalance of the oxidant-antioxidant system, infectious agents and activation of immune-competent cells seem to be essential as well [1, 5, 6]. Opie [7, 8] postulated almost one century ago that autodigestion has been induced by stone impaction at the ampulla of Vater leading to outflow obstruction of a common channel between the common bile duct and the pancreatic duct resulting in pancreatic necrosis.

Table 1. Causes of acute pancreatitis

Biliary tract disease
Ethyl alcohol abuse
Peptic ulcer
Trauma, surgery
Pregnancy (third trimester)
Vascular factors
Hyperlipoproteinemias (type I, IV, V)
Hypercalcemia (hyperparathyroidism, multiple myeloma)
Drugs (azathioprine, estrogens, corticosteroids, thiazides)
Hereditary pancreatitis
Pancreas divisum (?)
Infectious agents (bacterial, viral)
Methyl alcohol, *L*-asparaginase
Scorpion bites
Carcinoma of the pancreas, primary and metastatic
Organic solvents
Hypotensive shock
Endoscopic retrograde cholangiopancreaticography

This hypothesis, accepted for a long time, is now being challenged. There is no doubt that most attacks of pancreatitis due to gallstones are associated with the migration of a stone in the duodenum perhaps with transient delay in migration at the ampulla or with induction of ampullary edema. Gallstones are found in the stool of 85–95% of patients during an attack of acute biliary pancreatitis compared to only 10% in patients with gallstones but without pancreatitis [9, 10]. The incidence of common bile duct stones at the time of urgent operation after acute pancreatitis has been reported in 63–78% [11, 12, 15] by some but only in less than 33% by others [11–13]. Cystic ducts were larger in patients which suffered from acute pancreatitis and a larger number of small stones was found in these patients as well [11, 15]. However, in a prospective study, even in patients undergoing emergency operation, only in 6% of the patients was ampullary stone impaction found [16]. In addition, in experimental situations obstruction of the pancreatic duct alone usually induces only mild edema in contrast to necrotizing pancreatitis being followed after reflux of bile mixed with pancreatic juice [5]. The severity of necrosis and hemorrhage seems to be determined at the onset by the amount and concentration of bile salts reaching the acini, at least in animals [29]. Kelly and Wagner's data [17] supported this idea by findings in men. Progression of the disease seemed to be fixed from the onset independent of stone impaction. In a carefully conducted, prospective, randomized study, they demonstrated that edematous or hemorrhagic necrotizing pancreatitis can develop with or without impacted stones not being influenced by early surgical decompression, questioning somehow the hypothesis of autodigestion following stone impaction. Thus, although there is a definite association between acute pancreatitis and migration of gallstones, the role of ampullary obstruction by microcalculi or edema and the importance of persistence of stone impaction remains unclear.

There is some evidence that even the opposite, an open sphincter of Vater leading to duodenopancreatic reflux, might be of greater importance. The high incidence of pancreatic duct reflux during operative cholangiography in patients undergoing cholecystectomy after gallstone-associated pancreatitis is well known [11, 18]. This reflux is associated with a low common bile duct pressure [19]. In addition, patients with reflux had wider cystic and common bile ducts and multiple small stones in the gallbladder [18] supporting the hypothesis that gallstone migration is associated with reflux [20] which can induce pancreatitis. Pancreatitis may be caused by reflux of activating duodenal juice or bacterial toxins. This hypothesis has been supported by animal models as well [5]. Healthy people are protected against reflux from the duodenum [20]. In healthy people reflux to the common bile duct and to the pancreatic duct is rarely seen and bile and pancreatic juice are sterile under normal conditions. This is in accordance with the finding of a higher pressure in the pancreatic duct than in the common bile duct [20, 21]. Duct pressures are dependent on volume capacity, secretion rate and outlet resistance. During gallbladder contraction common bile duct pressure may exceed the pressure of the pancreatic duct in healthy people but reflux in the pancreatic duct seems to be unlikely due to the lower pressure in the duodenum and the cholecysto-sphincter of Odii reflex. The findings in patients with common bile duct stones are partially incongruent [20]. Gregg and Carr-Locke [22] observed an increased common bile duct pressure in patients with stones in the common bile duct which has been even higher than the pressure in the pancreatic duct supporting reflux in the pancreatic system in contrast to the situation in normals. This might be a factor in the pathogenesis of severe pancreatitis seen more often in patients with common bile duct stones. The function of the sphincter of Odii, however, may be of more importance but little is known about the functional activity of the different sphincter zones of the biliary and pancreatic duct and their inter-relationship in men especially in pancreatic disease. Motility disturbances of the sphincter may be secondary to initial stone passage. This observation of elevated pressure in the common bile duct in patients with common bile duct stones has not been found by others, however [27, 28]. In addition, the evaluation of 614 operative cholangiograms in patients undergoing cholecystectomy for biliary lithiasis did not show a significant correlation between the presence of common bile duct stone and bilio-pancreatic reflux [18].

Findings of reflux in the pancreatic duct, postulated sphincter dysfunction and of at least transient outflow obstructions lead to an unproven but intriguing hypothesis of gallstone-associated pancreatitis comprising different pathogenetic phases. First the impaction or the migration of a small gallstone through the ampulla induces edema and malfunction of the sphincter of Odii leading to bilio-pancreatic reflux. Reflux and obstruction might induce acute pancreatitis which can be aggravated by spasm and edema of the sphincter of Odii as well as by inflammation involving the peri-pancreatic duodenum. In the later phase, atony of the sphincter and the duodenum may form a duodeno-bilio-pancreatic cloaca as suggested by Arianoff [23]. A higher pressure in the common bile duct than in the pancreatic duct due to common bile duct stones will further increase bilio-pancreatic reflux perhaps aggravating pancreatitis thereby. This hypothesis would be in accordance with the theory of Neoptolemos [24], the data of whom suggested a relationship between persisting common bile duct stones and severity of pancreatitis. Bacterial content of the reflux as well as other factors [5, 25, 26] may play a crucial role in determination of the severity and the sequels as suggested by animal studies. Keynes [25] demonstrated the significance of bacterial enzymes causing membrane disturbances and hemorrhagic pancreatitis in dogs. Bacterial enzymes or toxins may trigger the release of inflammatory mediators from leukocytes and monocytes as well.

Surgery in Gallstone Pancreatitis

Acosta et al. [30] recommended in 1978 early surgery within 24–48 h in patients with gallstone pancreatitis. His uncontrolled data suggested that morbidity and mortality are reduced by this aggressive approach, but other again uncontrolled studies could not confirm these results. Ranson [31] observed a higher mortality in early operated patients. The patients of Ranson's group, however, suffered from much more severe pancreatitis than the patients in Acosta's study. Ranson's findings have been confirmed recently by a carefully conducted prospective study by Kelly and Wagner [32]. Early surgery (within 48 h after admission to the hospital) resulted in a morbidity of 30.1% and a mortality of 15.1% compared to 5.1 and 2.4%, respectively, in patients with delayed operation. Whereas the prognosis of patients with mild pancreatitis has not been affected by the time of surgery, the risk in patients with severe pancreatitis was unacceptably high. Congruous data have been found by Kim et al. [33]. According to the evaluation of 104 consecutive operations, it is not the timing of surgery for acute gallstone pancreatitis which seems to be crucial but the severity of the disease and the medical risk factors of the patients.

According to current knowledge early surgery should not be aimed for routinely in acute gallstone pancreatitis. However, there is agreement that cholecystectomy should be performed early after acute pancreatitis has resolved if the clinical risk is acceptable [34].

Sphincterotomy in Gallstone-Associated Pancreatitis

Despite not being conclusive, the theoretical data collected above suggest that obstruction of the sphincter of Odii by stone impaction may induce pancreatitis but does not determine the severity of disease. Early surgery to remove impacted common bile duct stones is of no benefit. Reflux of bile or duodenal content could be of much greater importance questioning the need for endoscopic sphincterotomy in patients with gallstone-associated pancreatitis. Theoretically, reflux could even be increased by sphincterotomy.

However, there are good arguments supporting early sphincterotomy: Independent of the pathophysiological mechanism of biliary pancreatitis, severe pancreatitis, complications in the course, and unfavorable outcome of biliary pancreatitis are seen more often in patients with common bile duct stones. Neoptolemos [24] suggested, therefore, as discussed above, that the initial attack of pancreatitis is induced by a stone which will pass into the duodenum during the acute attack in most of the patients leaving the pathogenetic mechanism open. Persisting common bile duct stones, however, shall be responsible for the severity of the disease perhaps due to the intermittent pancreatic duct obstruction caused by impaction of the stone in the sphincter followed by disimpaction back into the bile duct. On the other hand, common bile duct stones could influence sphincter motility and reflux in the pancreatic system as well.

Different clinical studies support sphincterotomy in patients with biliary pancreatitis. In a study of patients with idiopathic recurrent pancreatitis, surgically or endoscopically remediable conditions were looked for by ERCP and sometimes by manometry [4]. Despite the differences in pathology, long-term follow-up up to 3–4 years showed only a rare recurrence of pancreatitis in the dysmotility group and after operative accessory sphincteroplasty or endoscopic dilatation of the minor papilla in the pancreas divisum group. Despite the controversy on the significance of these entities the results are impressive and support the possible importance of sphincter dysfunction in the pathogenesis of pancreatitis and the role of sphincterotomy.

Several noncontrolled studies reported on the rapid improvement of gallstone pancreatitis after endoscopic sphincterotomy [35–41]. Keeping in mind the frequent spontaneous rapid improvement of biliary pancreatitis interpretation of these results is difficult. However, they prove that endoscopic papillotomy can be done with an acceptable risk even in acute pancreatitis. The complication rate has been low in all series (0–11%) with only few deaths (0–7.1%, average 2.1%). These results are congruent with a recent multicenter study with 284 patients [41]. The complication rate was not significantly higher than that reported for 1,000 consecutive patients treated by endoscopic sphincterotomy for common bile duct disease without pancreatitis [46]. ERCP and papillotomy has been done in most of these studies by experienced endoscopists, however.

Up to now only one prospective controlled study has been reported. Neoptolemos et al. [42] undertook a 4-year prospective randomized trial to assess the safety and efficacy of endoscopic sphincterotomy in acute gallstone pancreatitis. Of 223 patients 146 were suspected to have gallstone pancreatitis by sonography or biochemical parameters. Of these finally 121 were randomized to receive either conventional treatment or undergo ERCP within 72 h with endoscopic sphincterotomy and endoscopic stone extraction if common bile duct stones have been found. All endoscopies were performed by one highly skilled endoscopist. Patients have been stratified before to mild or severe disease according to a modification of the Glasgow criteria [42]. Cholangiography was successfully accomplished in 80% of patients with severe disease (25 patients) and in 94% of those with predicted mild attacks (34 patients). The results of this study from Leicester (UK) were quite interesting. Common bile duct stones were found in 63% of those with predicted severe disease but only in 26% with mild disease. In the conventionally treated group, only in 13% of the cases were common bile duct stones seen subsequently. Morbidity in patients with severe disease was 24% in the group with active evaluation compared to 61% in the conservatively treated patients. In addition, there was a significant reduction in hospital stay following urgent sphincterotomy in the group with severe disease (median 9.5 vs. 17 days) [11, 42]. There was a definite trend without statistical significance to a reduction in mortality as well with 1 death in the endoscopically evaluated group (2%) and 5 in the conservatively treated patients (8%). Results were the same if only patients with confirmed gallstones were evaluated. No benefit was shown for patients with mild disease but the complication rate was not higher in endoscopied patients either. This well-conducted study confirms again that ERCP and sphincterotomy can be performed safely by experienced hands in patients with acute pancreatitis. Exacerbation of pancreatitis or infection into devitalized pancreas has not been observed. The patients received cefuroxime prophylactically. One major drawback of the study is that finally only a few patients had papillotomy, exact data not have been presented. Results have not been analyzed accordingly most likely due to the too small number. That leaves the question of the value of urgent sphincterotomy in gallstone pancreatitis somewhat open. It also remains to be firmly established that the duration of lodgement of a stone in the common bile duct is related to the severity of pancreatitis. We hope that controlled studies under way in Germany [15] can answer these remaining problems better.

Endoscopic Sphincterotomy, an Unresolved Question?

Different studies have shown that an ERCP should be carried out if a positive cause of pancreatitis does not emerge [4, 43]. Neither ultrasound nor computer tomography can be relied upon to pick up all the patients with gallstones. The data presented above clearly demonstrate that experienced endoscopists can safely perform ERCP in acute pancreatitis. However, the importance and the timing of endoscopic papillotomy remains unknown. Present data strongly suggest that urgent endoscopy and papillotomy in cases of persisting common bile duct is of benefit despite that the pathophysiological rationale for it is unknown. However, this only seems to be true for patients with severe disease. Ideal ways to predict early prognosis using methods feasible even for district hospitals, especially in attacks due to gallstones, have unfortunately still not been found [44]. At the moment it may therefore be wise to perform urgent ERCP within a delay of 72 h but this may prove to be wrong in the near future. Sphincterotomy may prevent recurrence of pancreatitis not only by removal of the common bile duct stone but also by separation of the biliary system from the pancreatic duct. The main advantage of endoscopic sphincterotomy compared to surgery is its safety and easiness to be performed quickly by experienced endoscopists even in very ill patients.

However, we have to keep in mind that most of the common bile duct stones pass spontaneously without affecting the outcome. What will the long-term results in patients with unnecessarily destroyed papillary sphincters be? In contrast to surgical sphincteroplasties endoscopic sphincterotomy is, most of the time, incomplete [20]. Even after complete endoscopic sphincterotomy of the biliary sphincter, a distinct pancreatic sphincter remains functional [20, 22, 45] but pancreatic duct pressure is reduced [22]. This may prevent the creation of a bilio-duodeno-pancreatic cloaca and its possible dangerous sequelae. Long-term follow-up after endoscopic sphincterotomy of 1,050 patients in a multicenter study evaluating initially 9,041 patients from 25 centers showed restenosis in 3.1% and recurrence of stones in 5.8% but no cholangitis or pancreatitis [46].

Today, I suggest that every patient with gallstone pancreatitis and persisting common bile duct stone or absence of improvement within the first 48 h should be evaluated endoscopically and should undergo endoscopic papillotomy if a bile duct stone is found. To prevent further complications, early cholecystectomy after recovery of the acute attack should be performed during the same hospitalisation. However, lacking enough conclusive data this statement might be wrong tomorrow.

References

1 Geokas MC, Baltaxe HA, Banks PA, Silva J, Frey CF: Acute pancreatitis. Ann Intern Med 1985;103:86–100.
2 Norback I: Acute necrotizing pancreatitis after exposure to polychlorinated biphenyls. Ital J Gastroenterol 1987;19:278–279.
3 Celifarco N, Warschauer MD, Burakoff R: Metronidazole induced pancreatitis. Am J Gastroenterol 1989; 34:958–960.
4 Venu RP, Greenen JE, Hogan W, Stone J, Johnson GK, Soergel K: Idiopathic recurrent pancreatitis: An approach to diagnosis and treatment. Dig Dis Sci 1989;34:56–60.
5 McMahon MJ: Acute pancreatitis. Curr Opin Gastroenterol 1989;5: 693–700.
6 Gudgeon MA, Heath DI, Hurley P, Jehan IA, Patel G, Wilson C, Shenkin A, Austen BM, Imrie CW, Hermon Taylor J: Trypsinogen activation peptides assay in the early prediction of severity of acute pancreatitis. Lancet 1990;335:4–8.
7 Opie EL: The etiology of acute haemorrhagic pancreatitis. Johns Hopkins Hosp Bull 1901;121:182–188.
8 Opie EL: The relation of cholelithiasis to disease of the pancreas and to fat necrosis. Am J Med Sci 1901; 121:27–43.
9 Acosta JM, Ledesma CL: Gallstone migration as a cause of acute pancreatitis. N Engl J Med 1974;290:484–487.
10 Kelly TR, Serancy PE: Gallstone pancreatitis: The second time around. Surgery 1982;92:571–574.
11 Carr-Locke DL: Acute gallstone pancreatitis and endoscopic therapy. Endoscopy 1990;22:180–183.
12 Kelly TR: Gallstone pancreatitis. The timing of surgery. Surgery 1980; 88:345–350.
13 Mackie CR, Wood RAB, Preece PE, Cuschieri A: Surgical pathology at early elective operation for suspected acute gallstone pancreatitis: Preliminary report of a prospective trial. Br J Surg 1985;72:179–181.
14 Armstrong CP, Taylor TV, Jeacock J, Lucas S: The biliary tract in patients with acute gallstone pancreatitis. Br J Surg 1985;72:551.
15 Lankisch PG, Mahlke R, Lübbers H: Endoskopische Papillotomie als Frühmassnahme bei akuter Pankreatitis – eine kritische Einordnung der Indikation. Internist 1989;30: 725–729.
16 Stone HH, Fabian TC, Dunlop WE: Gallstone pancreatitis. Biliary tract pathology in relation to time of operation. Ann Surg 1981;194:305–312.
17 Elliott DW: Gallstone pancreatitis: When is the optimal time for intervention? Hepatology 1989;6:1022–1024.
18 Armstrong CP, Taylor TV: Pancreatic duct reflux and acute gallstone pancreatitis. Ann Surg 1986; 204:59–64.
19 Cuschieri A, Howell-Hughes J: Pancreatic reflux during operative choledochography. Br J Surg 1973;60: 933–936.
20 Funch-Jensen P: Sphincter of Oddi motility. Acta Chir Scand 1990; (suppl 553):1–35.
21 Carr-Locke DL, Gregg JA: Endoscopic manometry of pancreatic and biliary sphincter zones in man: Basal results in healthy volunteers. Dig Dis Sci 1981;26:7–15.
22 Gregg JA, Carr-Locke DL: Endoscopic pancreatic and biliary manometry in pancreatic, biliary, and papillary disease, and after endoscopic sphincterotomy and surgical sphincteroplasty. Gut 1984;25: 1247–1254.
23 Arianoff AA: Pancreatic duct reflux and acute pancreatitis; in Hollender LF (ed): Controversies in Acute Pancreatitis. Berlin, Springer, 1982, pp 7–8.
24 Neoptolemos JP: The theory of 'persisting' common bile duct stones in severe gallstone pancreatitis. Ann Royal Coll Surg Engl 1989;71:327–331.
25 Keynes WM: A non-pancreatic source of proteolytic enzyme amidase and bacteriology in experimental pancreatitis. Ann Surg 1980;191: 187–199.
26 Leading Article: Obstruction or reflux in gallstone associated acute pancreatitis? Lancet 1988;i:915–917.
27 Tanaka M, Ikeda S, Nakayama F: Non-operative measurement of pancreatic and common bile duct pressures with a micro transducer catheter and effects of duodenoscopic sphincterotomy. Dig Dis Sci 1981; 26:545–552.

28 Csendes A, Cruse A, Funch-Jensen P, Osler MJ, Ornsholt J, Andrup E: Pressure measurements in the biliary and pancreatic duct systems in controls and in patients with gallstones, previous cholecystectomy, or common bile duct stones. Gastroenterology 1979;77:1203–1210.
29 Elliott DW, Williams RD, Zollinger RM: Alterations in the pancreatic resistence to bile in the pathogenesis of acute pancreatitis. Ann Surg 1957;146:669–682.
30 Acosta JM, Prossie R, Galli OMR, Pelligini CA, Skinner DB: Early surgery for acute gallstone pancreatitis: evaluation of a systemic approach. Surgery 1978;83:367–371.
31 Ranson JH: The timing of biliary surgery in acute pancreatitis. Ann Surg 1979;189:654–657.
32 Kelly TR, Wagner DS: Gallstone pancreatitis: A prospective randomized trial of the timing of surgery. Surgery 1988;104:600–605.
33 Kim U, Shen HY, Bodner B: Timing of surgery for acute gallstone pancreatitis. Am J Surg 1988;156:393–396.
34 Beger HG: Akute Pankreatitis bei Choledocholithiasis – Papillotomie versus Operation. Chirurgischer Standpunkt. Z Gastroenterol 1985; 23:63–68.
35 Van Husen N: Akute Pankreatitis bei Choledocholithiasis – Papillotomie versus Operation. Z. Gastroenterologie 1985;23:58–62.
36 Classen M, Ossenberg W, Wurbs D, Dammermann R, Hagenmüller F: Pancreatitis: An indication for endoscopic papillotomy (abstract)? Endoscopy 1978;10:223.
37 Van der Spuy DS: Endoscopic sphincterotomy in the management of gallstone pancreatitis. Endoscopy 1981;13:25–26.
38 Kautz G, Kohans H, Keferstein RD, Bunte H: Zur Pathogenese und endoskopischen Therapie der akuten biliären Pankreatitis. Klinikarzt 1982;11:1202–1212.
39 Von Riemann RF, Lux G: Therapeutische Strategie bei der akuten Pankreatitis. Fortschr Med 1984; 102:179–182.
40 Rosseland AR, Solhaug JH: Early or delayed endoscopic papillotomy in gallstone pancreatitis. Ann Surg 1984;199:165–167.
41 Farkas IE, Tulassay Z, Papp J: Endoscopic sphincterotomy in acute biliary pancreatitis: Results of an international study (abstract). Digestion 1988;40:80.
42 Neoptolemos JP, Carr-Locke DL, London NJ, Bailey IA, James D, Fossard DP: Controlled trial of urgent endoscopic retrograde cholangiopancreatography and endoscopic sphincterotomy versus conservative treatment for acute pancreatitis due to gallstones. Lancet 1989;ii:979–983.
43 Schölmerich J, Gross V, Johanesson T, Brobmann G, Ruchauer K, Wimmer B, Gerock W, Farthmann EH: Detection of biliary origin of acute pancreatitis: comparison of laboratory tests, ultrasound, computed tomography and ERCP. Dig Dis Sci 1989;34:830–833.
44 McMahon MJ: Acute pancreatitis. Curr Opin Gastroenterol 1990;6: 757–762.
45 Funch-Jensen P, Kruse A, Ravusbaek J, Raundahl U: Manometric findings and therapeutic endoscopic procedures in patients with postcholecystectomy pain. Ital J Gastroenterol 1987;19:171–173.
46 Vaira D, D'Anna L, Ainley C, Dowsett J, Williams S, Baillie J, Cairns S, Croker J, Salmon P, Cotton P, Russel C, Hatfield A: Endoscopic sphincterotomy in 1,000 consecutive patients. Lancet 1989;ii:431–433.

Dig Dis 1992;10:326–329

Christoph Beglinger

Division of Gastroenterology,
University Hospital, Basel,
Switzerland

Relevant Aspects of Physiology in Chronic Pancreatitis

Key Words
Cholinergic system
Cholecystokinin
Secretin

Abstract
Specific points of physiology which are relevant for the understanding and management of chronic pancreatitis are focussed on. First, the regulatory factors of exocrine pancreatic secretion are described, discussing the role of the cholinergic system and of the classical gut hormones cholecystokinin and secretin. The association of upper gastrointestinal dysfunctions with a disturbed exocrine pancreatic response is also dealt with. Lastly, these changes are related to clinical consequences such as maldigestion or malabsorption.

Introduction

The past decade has brought some remarkable advances in our knowledge about pancreatic physiology. However, little information is still available about many basic aspects of human pancreatic function because of the technical difficulties involved in collecting pure pancreatic juice from human subjects. This applies in particular to patients with chronic pancreatitis where only fragmental information is present on the regulation of pancreatic exocrine secretion. This chapter intends to illustrate specific points of physiology which are relevant for the understanding of chronic pancreatitis.

Functions of the Exocrine Pancreas

The major function of the exocrine pancreas involves the secretion of a bicarbonate-rich fluid and digestive enzymes into the duodenum, thereby playing a decisive role in the breakdown of food. The bicarbonate-rich fluid serves to neutralize gastric acid, a function which contributes to the homeostasis of the small intestinal 'milieu intérieur'. This in turn protects the duodenal mucosa against damage from gastric acid, but also provides the optimal conditions for cellular growth of the mucosa of the small intestine. The small intestinal homeostasis is furthermore essential to provide a functional pH value for the

Christoph Beglinger, MD
Division of Gastroenterology
University Hospital
CH–4031 Basel (Switzerland)

© 1992
S. Karger AG, Basel
0257–2753/92/
0106–0326$2.75/0

action of pancreatic digestive enzymes, brush-border enzymes and to keep bile salts in a soluble, dissociated form [1].

Chronic pancreatitis leads to a primary deficit in pancreatic bicarbonate secretion, but it is not clear yet whether this reduction in bicarbonate secretion has any negative consequences which are of clinical relevance [2].

A decreased pancreatic enzyme secretion on the other hand has clearly important negative consequences such as a malabsorption syndrome. This is a direct consequence of decreased intraluminal hydrolysis of food components with consequent caloric deficit, vitamin deficiencies, and fatty acid-induced diarrhea. It has to be stressed that more than 75–80% of the exocrine tissue have to be destroyed before a pancreatic enzyme insufficiency becomes clinically relevant [3].

Pancreatic Response to a Meal

Digestive Enzymes

About 90% of the exocrine pancreas consists of acinar cells primarily secreting enzymes for digestive functions. Enzymes are secreted by exocytosis and most of them are secreted as proenzymes which are enzymatically inert [4]. Only when the inactive precursor reaches the duodenal lumen, does an activating process begin. Trypsinogen is converted enzymatically into trypsin by the intestinal brush-border enzyme enterokinase. In turn, active trypsin converts other proenzymes into their active forms. The pancreatic proteases hydrolyze the peptide bonds of the protein components of food. The end products of these processes are mainly oligopeptides composed of 6 amino acid residues or less and some free amino acids [5]. Lipolysis results from activation of lipolytic enzymes and their action on fat entering the duodenum. In the intestinal lumen, the activated colipase binds to the surface of triglycerides allowing the lipase to gain access to its substrate [5]. Pancreatic lipase hydrolyzes triglycerides to monoglycerides and fatty acids. These breakdown products have a very low solubility in water, but are easily soluble in bile salt micelles which are necessary for absorption. In addition to lipase, the pancreas secretes cholesterol esterase, which hydrolyzes the ester bonds to yield free cholesterol, and phospholipases, which split lecithin to lysolecithins and free fatty acids. Digestion of starch by pancreatic amylase is a continuation of the breakdown process, started in the mouth by the activation of salivary amylase. The final results of the amylases on starch are di- or trisaccharides and alpha-limit dextrins [6].

Weight loss and steatorrhea are regular signs of severe chronic pancreatitis; they are indicative for maldigestion as a result of a reduction in the secretion of pancreatic digestive enzymes. When steatorrhea is present, pancreatic lipase output has decreased to less than 10% [3, 7]. It is seen in at least 1/3 of patients with chronic pancreatitis, but may reach a much higher percentage when patients are followed up for a longer period of time [8].

Pancreatic Response to a Meal

Food-stimulated pancreatic secretion is classically divided into 3 phases: cephalic, gastric, and intestinal. The 3 phases overlap and probably interact with each other. Little is known about the integrated pancreatic response to a meal. This is partly due to the technical difficulties and limitations involved in obtaining quantitative information on the postprandial secretion in man [9]. The only feasible approach to assess the pancreatic response to a meal in humans is a marker perfusion technique, which entails positioning of a multilumen tube in the small intestine to sample duodenal contents under perfusion of a nonabsorbable marker to calculate total secretory output. The pancreatic bicarbonate response after meal intake can, however, not be quantified with this technique, because bicarbonate in duodenal contents is immediately neutralized by incoming gastric acid and food components. Therefore, no exact information is available with respect to postprandial pancreatic bicarbonate secretion in healthy subjects and patients with chronic pancreatitis. Only a few studies have measured the pancreatic enzyme response after meal intake in humans. The enzyme response to a solid meal has been shown to be more prolonged than the response to a nutritionally equivalent liquid meal [10]. The secretory response to a liquid meal averages 50–60% of maximal capacity in normal subjects, raising the question whether the magnitude of pancreatic secretion in response to a meal is constant or whether it reflects a changing demand for digestion [11]. A recent study suggests that different caloric loads of a liquid meal induce different pancreatic enzyme responses [12].

Regulatory Factors

At the beginning of the century, Pavlow [13] suggested that the pancreas was exclusively controlled by neural mechanisms [13]. Later on, secretin and cholecystokinin were discovered, which prompted some authors to proclaim that the nervous regulation is 'superfluous and improbable' [14]. At present, it is clear that the cholinergic system is of crucial importance in regulating exocrine pancreatic secretion with cholecystokinin and secretin modifying the response [12]. Whether excess concentrations of CCK or deficiency of secretin levels have any role in the pathogenesis of chronic pancreatitis is a highly debated topic with little experimental support for these hypotheses [15, 16].

Association of Altered Gastrointestinal Functions with Disturbed Exocrine Pancreatic Secretion

As noted before, pancreatic enzymes are normally secreted in excess. In chronic pancreatitis, it normally takes several years for severe exocrine pancreatic insufficiency to develop, but lipase secretion is more rapidly impaired than the secretion of proteolytic enzymes [17], because lipase in the intestinal lumen is more fragile than the other enzymes. Lipase is easily inactivated by acidic pH and digested by proteolytic enzymes.

In patients with severe pancreatic insufficiency, duodenal pH appears to be in the normal range of pH 5–6 in the early postprandial phase, but is abnormally low (below pH 4) in the late postprandial period. This low intraduodenal pH is probably due to decreased bicarbonate secretion from the pancreas, but it has 2 important consequences: (1) a low pH inactivates pancreatic lipase activity; (2) a low pH promotes precipitation of bile acids. Both factors reduce lipid digestion, thus further increasing fat malabsorption and steatorrhea [18]. Raising intraduodenal pH to normal values by giving antisecretory drugs which reduce gastric acid secretion, has been reported to prevent bile acid precipitation, thus improving lipid digestion [18]. Rapid gastric emptying of liquid fatty meals has been reported in patients with chronic pancreatic insufficiency, but most available evidence suggests that the rate of gastric emptying is normal in chronic pancreatitis. Thus, an impaired gastric emptying rate is unlikely to be of physiological importance in the patients with chronic exocrine pancreatic insufficiency.

Conclusion

The pancreatic enzymes are essential for normal digestion and subsequent absorption of food. A decreased pancreatic secretory response due to chronic pancreatitis causes maldigestion of food components and leads to malabsorption. The present chapter summarizes the main aspects of normal physiology of exocrine pancreatic secretion and relates them to changes in pancreatic insufficiency.

Acknowledgements

The author is supported by a grant of the Swiss National Science Foundation (grant 3.890-0.88).

The author thanks Carita Frei for editorial assistance and typing the manuscript.

References

1 Solomon TE: Control of exocrine pancreatic secretion; in Johnson LR (ed): Physiology of the Gastrointestinal Tract, ed 2. New York, Raven Press, 1987, pp 1173–1207.

2 Schulze S, Thorsgaard Pedersen N, Jørgensen MJ, Møllmann KM, Rune SJ: Association between duodenal bulb ulceration and reduced exocrine pancreatic function. Gut 1983;24;781–783.

3 DiMagno EP, Go VLW, Summerskill WHJ: Relations between pancreatic enzyme outputs and malabsorption in severe pancreatic insufficiency. N Engl J Med 1973;288: 813–815.

4 Scheele G: Cellular processing of proteins in the exocrine pancreas; in Go VLW, Gardner JD, Brooks FP, Lebenthal E, DiMagno EP, Scheele GA (eds): The Exocrine Pancreas: Biology, Pathobiology, and Diseases. New York, Raven Press, 1986, pp 69–85.

5 Rinderknecht H: Pancreatic secretory enzymes; in Go VLW, Gardner JD, Brooks FP, Lebenthal E, DiMagno EP, Scheele GA (eds): The Exocrine Pancreas: Biology, Pathobiology, and Diseases. New York, Raven Press, 1986, pp 163–183.

6 Beck IT: The role of pancreatic enzymes in digestion. Am J Clin Nutr 1973;26:311–325.

7 Gyr NE: Tests of Exocrine Pancreatic Function. Bern, Huber, 1975.

8 Ammann RW, Akovbiantz A, Largiader F, Schueler G: Course and outcome of chronic pancreatitis. Longitudinal study of a mixed medical-surgical series of 245 patients. Gastroenterology 1984;86:820–828.

9 Adler G, Beglinger C: Hormones as regulators of pancreatic secretion in man. Eur J Clin Invest 1990;(suppl 1)20:S27–S32.

10 Malagelada JR, Go VLW, Summerskill WHJ: Different gastric, pancreatic, and biliary responses to solid-liquid or homogenized meals. Dig Dis Sci 1979;24:101–110.

11 Beglinger C, Fried M, Whitehouse O, Jansen JB, Lamers CB, Gyr K: Pancreatic enzyme response to a liquid meal and to hormonal stimulation. Correlation with plasma secretin and cholecystokinin levels. J Clin Invest 1985;75:1471–1476.

12 Adler G, Beglinger C, Braun U, Reinshagen M, Koop I, Schafmayer A, Rovati L, Arnold R: Interaction of the cholinergic system and cholecystokinin in the regulation of endogenous and exogenous stimulation of pancreatic secretion in humans. Gastroenterology 1991;100: 537–543.

13 Pavlow IP: The Work of the Digestive Glands (translated by Thompson WT). London, Griffin, 1902.

14 Bayliss W, Starling EH: Mechanism of pancreatic secretion. J Physiol (Lond) 1902;28:325–353.

15 Owyang C, Scarpello JH, Vinik AI: Correlation between pancreatic enzyme secretion and plasma concentration of human pancreatic polypeptide in health and in chronic pancreatitis. Gastroenterology 1982;83:55–62.

16 Mössner J, Wresky HP, Kestel W, Zeeh J, Regner U, Fischbach W: Influence of treatment with pancreatic extracts on pancreatic enzyme secretion. Gut 1989;30:1143–1149.

17 Regan PT, Malagelada JR, DiMagno EP, Go VLW: Postprandial gastric function in pancreatic insufficiency. Gut 1979;20:249–254.

18 Regan PT, Malagelada JR, DiMagno EP, Go VLW: Reduced intraluminal bile acid concentrations and fat maldigestion in pancreatic insufficiency: Correction by treatment. Gastroenterology 1979;77: 285–289.

Dig Dis 1992;10:330–334

P. Meyer[a]
P.A. Clavien[a]
J. Robert[a]
H. Hauser[b]
A. Rohner[a]

[a] Digestive Surgery,
Department of Surgery, and
[b] Department of Radiology,
University Hospital of Geneva,
Switzerland

Role of Imaging Technics in the Classification of Acute Pancreatitis

Key Words
Acute pancreatitis
Computed tomography
Prognostic factors

Abstract

This paper is a review of some aspects of acute pancreatitis (AP) (definition criteria, outcome, and prognostic factors) and a reminder of the invaluable contribution of computed tomography (CT) in confirming the diagnosis of AP, distinguishing between edematous and necrotizing forms, and in providing prognostic information via detection of possible extrapancreatic spreads (EPS). The Geneva experience (510 cases of AP over a 9-year period) has shown that no fatalities occurred when no EPS were found on CT performed within 48 h of admission; mortality was 1.5% in the case of 1 or 2 EPS and 19% in the case of 3 EPS or more.

Prognostic uncertainty of acute pancreatitis (AP) upon admission can result in inappropriate treatment with some cases being either under- or overtreated.

Numerous biological and morphological criteria have been devised to differentiate between benign and severe cases of AP. In the last 10 years, CT has supplanted conventional radiology and is now considered as the most sensitive imaging modality for patients suspected of having AP [1–8].

The role of early contrast-enhanced CT (CE-CT) within 48 h in the diagnosis, classification and prognosis of AP was prospectively studied in a series of 510 consecutive cases between 1980 and 1988 [9].

Clinical and Histological Background

Two types of AP can be recognized on an anatomical basis. 'Acute edematous pancreatitis' (AEP) is characterized by interstitial

P. Meyer, MD
Digestive Surgery
University Hospital of Geneva
CH–1211 Geneva 4 (Switzerland)

© 1992
S. Karger AG, Basel
0257–2753/92/
0106–0330$2.75/0

edema within the gland which can extend to the peri-pancreatic fat. 'Necrotizing AP' (NAP) has necrosis within the pancreas and/or the peri-pancreatic fat and is encountered in 8–32% of the cases [9, 10]. These two anatomical entities appear in the Marseilles Classifications [11, 12] and have quite distinct clinical courses. AEP usually follows a light course (LAP), except if severe health conditions exist prior to the bout of AP. On the contrary, most NAP are associated with complications resulting in severe (SAP) or fatal (FAP) outcome. Sixty percent of the cases of NAP develop septic problems [10] which are the main factor of mortality: 80% [13].

Frey and Beger recently suggested that infection of necrosis could occur in two fashions and that prognosis was worse in precocious infection (within 10 days) than in late infection (from 3 to 5 weeks) [13, 14].

Adequate managment of AP thus depends on the following: a correct diagnosis, differentiation between AEP and NAP, and early identification of NAP with infected necrosis.

Diagnosis of AP

As defined by the Cambridge Symposium [15], the diagnosis of AP relies on a combination of hyperamylasemia and abdominal pain. This relationship, however, is at fault in some 20% of cases inasmuch as diagnostic levels of amylase are arbitrarily chosen and that more than 200 techniques of amylase determinations have been described so far [16–18]. Thus, in the absence of any highly specific laboratory test, CT scan appears as the gold standard in the diagnosis of AP, especially for prospective studies [2, 3, 5, 16, 19]. CT scan adequately evaluates the pancreas and adjacent retroperitoneal structures in almost all individuals [20], while ultrasound is usually helpless when bowel gas distension is present [21].

The normal pancreas appears as sharply defined with a smooth contour or a slightly undulating acinar configuration. The fatty retroperitoneal space is homogeneously low in density. To enhance visualization of the gland, intravenous administration of contrast media is given whenever possible: the normal pancreas appears as a homogeneously enhanced structure.

A wide variety of CT findings have been described in AP: diffuse or segmental enlargement of the gland, ill-defined margins [1, 2, 6, 8, 22, 23], abnormal parenchymal enhancement [2, 6], loss of peripancreatic tissue planes [1, 2, 6, 8, 22, 23], intraperitoneal or retroperitoneal fluid collections [1, 6, 23], and thickening of the peripancreatic fascia [1, 6, 23].

CT scan was systematically performed at our institution within 48 h of admission in all patients suspected of having AP, i.e. with continuous upper abdominal pain compatible with a pancreatic origin regardless of amylase values obtained on admission (i.e. even when this enzyme was within normal values) [6, 9]. A previous report from our institution showed a 99% sensitivity and a 100% specificity for CE-CT in the diagnostic of 177 consecutive cases AP [6].

Diagnosis of Pancreatic Necrosis

Physical signs such as fever higher than 38 °C, abdominal distension or guarding, occlusion or abdominal masses are not necessarily correlated with pancreatic and/or extrapancreatic necrosis [24].

The following biological parameters have been credited for their prognostic value: albumin [25], methemalbumin [26], ribonuclease [27], phospholipase A2 [28], antiproteases such as α_1-antitrypsin and α_2-macroglobulin [29, 30], C3 and C4 fractions of complement [30, 31].

Mayer et al. [32] recently wrote that CRP greater than 75 mg/100 ml is found in severe cases of AP, and Buchler et al. [30] reported a 95% sensitivity when CRP was above 100 mg/100 ml. These biological parameters, however, cannot foretell early infection of necrosis.

There are still other indexes of gravity in AP: McMahon et al. [33] used the amount and color of ascites and/or peritoneal lavage. We compared determinations of amylase and lipase in serum and peritoneal fluid upon admission; there was a tendency for AP to be more severe when peritoneal enzyme concentrations exceeded those found in blood; this enzymatic score also bore a direct correlation with the presence of extrapancreatic spreads [34].

Prognosis via CT Scan

It has been suggested that a normal pancreas or retroperitoneal space on CT can exclude severe AP [3, 7, 8, 35, 36]. Hill et al. [2] correlated the initial CT findings with edematous or necrotizing AP.

Severity of the disease can be assessed either by estimating the presence and degree of pancreatic and peripancreatic inflammation and fluid accumulation [8, 37, 38], or by detecting the presence and extent of pancreatic necrosis by early CE-CT [6, 30, 39–42]. The main differences in estimating the severity of AP rely on the degree of contrast-enhancement of the pancreatic parenchyma [40], the quantification of pancreatic necrosis in percent of the entire gland [39], or on the presence and number of extrapancreatic phlegmonous spreads [6].

Phlegmonous spreads defined as necrotic tissue (intra- or extrapancreatic) are associated with changes in hemodynamics and vascular permeability [43–46] and can thus be detected by CE-CT [6].

Table. 1. Hospital course in terms of CT grading

CT criteria	Recording evolution, our series, %		
	LAP	SAP	FAP
CT1	89.3	10.6	0[1]
CT2	57.5	41	1.5[1]
CT3	22	59	19

[1] After exclusion of patients with severe health conditions prior to AP which contraindicated surgery or even percutaneous lavage alone.

The problem of the predictive value of these indicators of severity is evidenced by the fact that while most patients with pancreatic necrosis also have extensive extrapancreatic phlegmons, sometimes minimal peripancreatic changes may be seen in some of these patients [1, 6].

Conversely, marked extrapancreatic spreads are not necessarily associated with extensive pancreatic necrosis [6, 39, 42]. Finally, pancreatic necrosis may be absent initially and develop later on [39].

In our series of 501 consecutive patients with nonrecurrent AP evidenced by CE-CT within 48 h of admission [9], phlegmonous spreads served as the basis of a CT-grading system with three groups [6]: (group 1): no phlegmonous extrapancreatic spread; (group 2): phlegmonous extrapancreatic spreads in one or two areas; (group 3): phlegmonous extrapancreatic spreads in three areas or more.

Extrapancreatic spreads most commonly encountered are represented in figure 1.

These 3 CT groups were matched to 3 clinical groups (table 1). Clinical course was retrospectively defined: (1) the first group consisted of fatal AP (FAP); (2) the second group corresponded to severe AP (SAP) and consisted of patients who had one or more com-

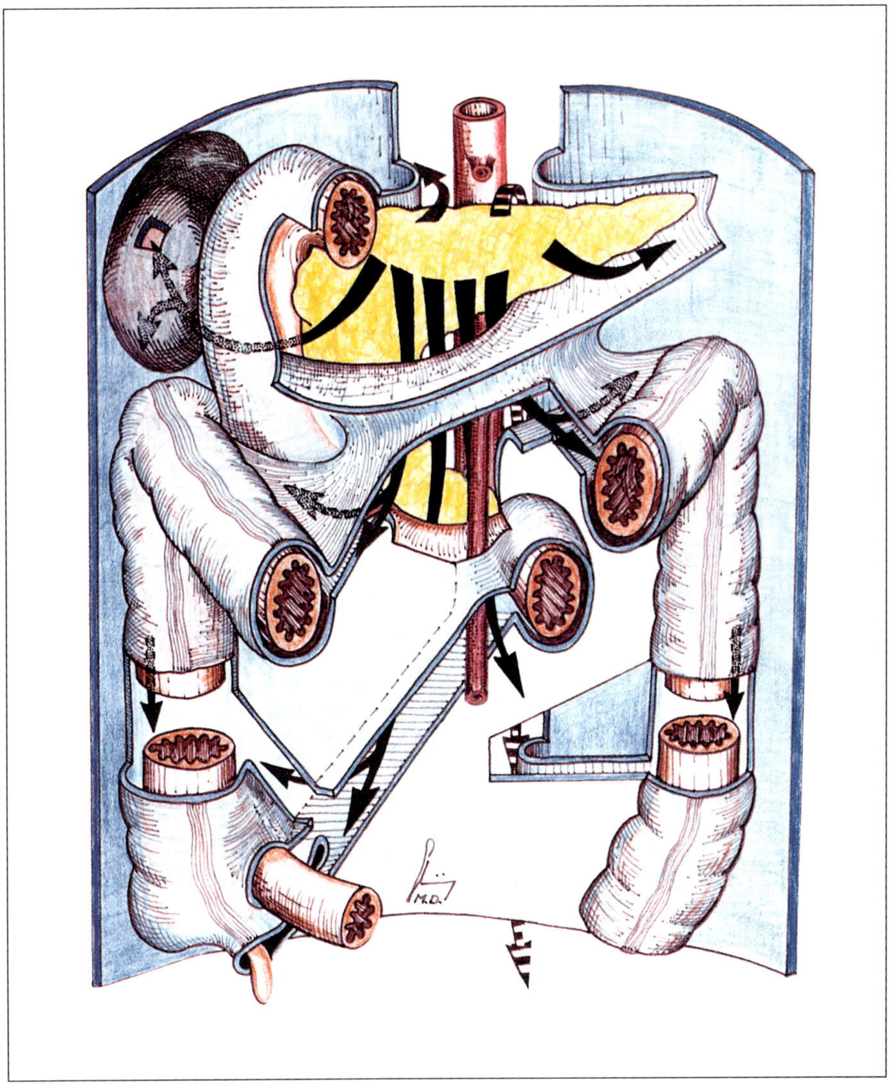

Fig. 1. Main extrapancreatic spreads (edema or necrosis).

plications, and/or required intensive care, and/or had hospital stays longer than 20 days; (3) the third group consisted of AP without any complication nor intensive care, and hospital stays shorter than 20 days (light AP, LAP).

According to this classification, there were no fatalities when no extrapancreatic necrotic spreads were found (CT group 1); within CT group 1, 90% of patients had benign clinical courses, whereas only 10% had severe pancreatitis, the latter consisting of noninfected pseudocysts which all resolved spontaneously without any treatment. On the contrary, when there were 3 extrapancreatic necrotic spreads or more (CT group 3), 78% of cases were severe (19% fatal) and only 22% benign. Finally, within the CT group 2, approximately one bout of AP out of two was severe with a 1.5% mortality [9].

In conclusion, any patient suspected of having AP should have a CT scan within 48 h of admission, since this exam can confirm the diagnosis of AP and avoid costly exacting measures if AP is edematous only.

In case of necrotizing AP, percutaneous aspiration of necrosis for bacteriological examination should be performed only in case of systemic repercussions such as respiratory, renal, or cardiovascular insufficiencies.

The other advantage of CE-CT is that it can detect other abdominal or retroperitoneal pathologies, should the pancreas be normal.

References

1 Balthazar EJ: CT-diagnosis and staging of acute pancreatitis. Radiol Clin North Am 1989;27:19–37.
2 Hill MC, Barkin J, Isikoff MB, et al: Acute pancreatitis: Clinical vs. CT findings. AJR 1982;139:263–269.
3 Jeffrey RB, Federle MP, Cello JP, et al: Early computed tomographic scanning in acute severe pancreatitis. Surg Gynecol Obstet 1982;154: 170–174.
4 Mendez G Jr, Isikoff MB, Hill MC: CT of pancreatitis: Interim assessment. AJR 1980;135:463–469.
5 Silverstein W, Isikoff MB, Hill MC, et al: Diagnostic imaging of acute pancreatitis: prospective study using CT and sonography. AJR 1981;137: 497–502.
6 Clavien PA, Hauser H, Meyer P, et al: Value of contrast-enhanced computerized tomography in the early diagnosis and prognosis of acute pancreatitis. Am J Surg 1988;155: 457–466.
7 Ranson JHC, Balthazar E, Caccavale R, et al: Computed tomography and the prediction of pancreatic abscess in acute pancreatitis. Ann Surg 1985;201:656–665.
8 Nordestgaard AG, Wilson SE, William RA: Early computerized tomography as a predictor of outcome in acute pancreatitis. Am J Surg 1986;152:127–130.
9 Meyer P: La pancréatite aiguë; thèse de Privat-Docent. Université de Genève, Août, 1989.
10 Beger HG, Block S, Bittner R: The significance of bacterial infection in acute pancreatitis; in Beger HG, Büchler M (eds): Acute Pancreatitis. Berlin, Springer, 1987, pp 79–80.
11 Sarles H: Proposal adopted unanimously by the participants of the Symposium on Pancreatitis at Marseille – 1963 –. Bibl Gastroenterol (Basel) 1965;7:7.
12 Gyr KE, Singer MV, Sarles H: Pancreatitis: Concepts and Classification; in Gyr KE, Singer MV, Sarles H (eds): Proceedings of the Second International Symposium of the Classification of Pancreatitis. Marseille, France, March 28–30. Amsterdam, Elsevier, 1984, pp 1–450.
13 Frey CF, Bradley EL III, Beger HG: Progress in acute pancreatitis. Surg Gynecol Obstet 1988;167:282–286.
14 Beger HG, Bittner R, Block S, et al: Bacterial contamination of pancreatic necrosis. Gastroenterology 1986;91:433–438.
15 Sarner M, Cotton PB: Classification of pancreatitis. Gut 1984;25:756–759.
16 Clavien PA, Robert J; Meyer P, et al: Acute pancreatitis and normoamylasemia. Ann Surg 1989;210: 614–620.
17 Salt WB, Schenker S: Amylase – its clinical significance: A review of the literature. Medicine 1976;55:269–289.
18 Ying Foo A, Rosalki SB: Measurement of plasma amylase activity. Ann Clin Biochem 1986;23:624–637.
19 Moossa AR: Diagnostic tests and procedures in acute pancreatitis. N Engl J Med 1984;311:639–643.
20 Neff CC, Ferrucci JT Jr: Pancreatitis. Surg Clin North Am 1984;64: 23–36.
21 Agarwal N, Pitchumoni CS, Sivaprasad AV: Evaluating tests for acute pancreatitis. Am J Gastroenterol 1990;85:356–366.

22 Becker H, Gahbauer H, Horn J, et al: Korrelation klinischer und computertomographischer Befunde für die Therapie und Prognose der akuten Pankreatitis. Chirurgie 1985;56:386–392.
23 McNeil BJ, Keeler E, Adelstein SJ: Primer on certain elements of medical decision making. N Engl J Med 1975;293:211–215.
24 Nordback I, Pessi T, Auvinen O, et al: Determination of necrosis in necrotizing pancreatitis. Br J Surg 1985;72:225–227.
25 Jacobs ML, Daggett WM, Civetta JM, et al: Acute pancreatitis: Analysis of factors influencing survival. Ann Surg 1977;185:43–46.
26 Winstone NE: Methaemalbumine in acute pancreatitis. Br J Surg 1965; 52:804–808.
27 Warshaw AL, Lee KH: Serum ribonuclease elevation and pancreatic necrosis in acute pancreatitis. Surgery 1979;86:227–234.
28 Schroder T, Kivilaakso E, Kinnunen PKJ, et al: Serum phospholipase A2 in human acute pancreatitis. Scand J Gastroenterol 1980;15: 633–636.
29 McMahon MJ, Bowen M, Mayer AD, et al: Relationship of alpha-2-macroglobuline and other antiprotease to the clinical features of acute pancreatitis. Am J Surg 1984;147: 164–170.
30 Buchler M, Malfertheiner P, Beger HG: Correlation of imaging procedures, biochemical parameters, and clinical stage in acute pancreatitis; in Malfertheiner P, Ditschuneit H, (eds): Diagnostic Procedures in Pancreatic Disease. Berlin, Springer, 1986, pp 123–129.
31 Foulis AK, Murray WR, Galloway D, et al: Endotoxaemia and complement activation in acute pancreatitis in man. Gut 1982;23:661–665.
32 Mayer AD, McMahon MJ, Bowen M, et al: C-reactive protein: An aid to assessment and monitoring of acute pancreatitis. J Clin Pathol 1984;37:207–211.
33 McMahon MJ, Pickford IR, Playforth MJ: Early prediction of severity of acute pancreatitis using peritoneal lavage. Acta Chir Scand 1980; 146:171–175.
34 Robert JH, Meyer P, Rohner A: Can serum and peritoneal amylase and lipase determinations help in the early prognosis of acute pancreatitis? Ann Surg 1986;203:163–168.
35 Frija J, Anabou A, Viandier A, et al: Computed tomography of severe acute pancreatitis. J Radiol 1983; 64:483–488.
36 Damman HG, Grabbe E, Runge M: Computed tomography and acute pancreatitis. Lancet 1980;ii:860.
37 Balthazar EJ, Ranson JHC, Naidich DP, et al: Acute pancreatitis: Prognostic value of CT. Radiology 1985; 156:767–772.
38 Vernacchia FS, Jeffrey RB Jr, Federle MP, et al: Pancreatic abscess: Predictive value of early abdominal CT. Radiology 1987;162:435–438.
39 Beger HG, Maier W, Block S, et al: How do imaging methods influence the surgical strategy in acute pancreatitis?; in Malfertheiner P, Ditschuneit H (eds): Diagnostic Procedures in Pancreatic Disease. Berlin, Springer, 1986, pp 54–60.
40 Kivisaari L, Kalevi S, Standertskjold-Nordenstamm CG, et al: A new method for the diagnosis of acute hemorrhagic-necrotizing pancreatitis using constrast-enhanced CT. Gastrointest Radiol 1984;9:27–30.
41 Kivisaari L, Somer K, Standertskjold-Nordenstam CG, et al: Early detection of acute fulminant pancreatitis by contrast enhanced computed tomography. Scand J Gastroenterol 1983;18:39–41.
42 Maier W: Grading of acute pancreatitis computed tomography morphology; in Malfertheiner P, Ditschuneit H (eds): Diagnostic Procedures in Pancreatic Disease. Berlin, Springer, 1986, pp 44–53.
43 Warshaw AL: Inflammatory masses following acute pancreatitis. Surg Clin North Am 1975;54:621–636.
44 Kormano M; in Felix R, Kazner E, Wegener OH (eds): Contrast Media in Computed Tomography. Amsterdam, Excerpta Medica, 1981, pp 38–45.
45 Carey L: Extra-abdominal manifestations of acute pancreatitis. Surgery 1979;86:337–342.
46 Donaldson LA, Schenk WG Jr: The effect of trasylol and vasopressin on experimental pancreatitis. Surg Gynecol Obstet 1980;15:657–669.

Dig Dis 1992;10:335–344

R. Muench

Department of Medicine,
University Hospital, Zurich,
Switzerland

Etiology and Natural History of Chronic Pancreatitis

Key Words
Chronic pancreatitis
Etiology
Natural history

Abstract
Chronic pancreatitis (CP) is a rare but serious disease with high morbidity and mortality. Its exact etiology remains uncertain, but several associated conditions have been identified. Geographical distribution of CP can be linked to alcoholism, especially in countries with high-protein, high-fat diets. In Afro-Asiatic countries with protein malnutrition, however, CP is frequently observed in children and young nonalcoholic adults from the poorest segments of these societies. To analyze the natural history of CP, besides etiology three additional main factors have to be considered, namely clinical pattern and therapy (surgery), pancreatic function (endocrine and exocrine), and morphology. During progress of the disease clinical picture, morphology and pancreatic function have typical correlative changes. Basically, from this viewpoint, three typical models of the disease can be distinguished: (1) early stage of uncomplicated CP; (2) late stage of uncomplicated CP, and (3) complicated CP, a disease stage which is characterised by local complications (chiefly pseudocysts and duct obstruction). The main concept of the natural history of CP bases on the thesis that CP burns itself out with spontaneous relief of pain, i.e. persistent freedom from pain occurs parallel with severe pancreatic dysfunction in the late stage of the disease. In the clinical picture and long-term course, nonalcoholic CP differs in certain essential respects from alcoholic CP; however, the two forms do not differ essentially as regards mortality and survival.

R. Muench, MD
Department of Medicine
University Hospital
CH–8091 Zurich (Switzerland)

© 1992
S. Karger AG, Basel
0257–2753/92/
0106–0335$2.75/0

Introduction

The first comprehensive description of chronic pancreatitis (CP) by Comfort et al. [1] in 1946 was mainly based on clinical observations, surgical and pathological findings. Development of pancreatic function tests and more recently advent of imaging techniques in the form of ERCP, ultrasound and computer tomography have increased our knowledge of this disease. An overview of the different clinical pictures associated with CP is given in table 1.

With regard to the pathophysiology, three major pathogenetic mechanisms are of special importance for the development of CP: (1) Epidemiological data support the causal relationship between alcohol consumption and CP and point toward an adjuvant role for genetic, dietary and environmental factors. (2) Because nonalcoholic pancreatitis in young people is frequent in Afro-Asian countries where malnutrition is prevalent, protein deprivation has been suggested as a possible cause. (3) Sophisticated methods like endoscopy and manometry enable us to study the pressure of the sphincter of Oddi and help to clarify the role of motility disorders of the sphincter of Oddi in CP.

Table 1. Etiology of CP

1	Alcohol
2	Idiopathic
	Juvenile CP
	Senile CP
3	Malnutrition
4	Rare causes
	Hereditary
	Metabolic
	Biliary disease?
	Congenital abnormalities
	Drugs (analgetica)
	Trauma
	Renal transplantation

Pathogenesis of Chronic Pancratitis

Alcohol

Alcohol is the predominant etiological factor in CP, especially in Europe and the USA. The number of cases of CP related to alcohol abuse varies from 36 to 85% [2–13]. The incidence of CP in the area of Zurich, Switzerland, has been evaluated repeatedly over the last 20 years [2, 9, 14]. Between 1958 and 1982, the incidence increased from 0.15 to 1.64 per 100,000 (table 2). This increase can be attributed mainly to the abuse of alcohol because the incidence of nonalcoholic CP remained remarkably stable over the past two decades. Similar results could be obtained in Copenhagen county in the period from 1970 to 1979 where a marked increase in alcohol consumption in Denmark after the second world war was paralleled by a significant increase in the incidence rate of CP [13]. As shown by a numer of studies [6, 10, 15–17], alcohol consumption was significantly higher in patients with CP than in controls. Sarles et al. [17] estimated a mean consumption of 150–175 g of pure alcohol per day associated with a diet significantly richer in proteins and fat. The same group was later able to demonstrate a linear relationship between alcohol consumption and the logarithmic risk for CP [18]. However, no statistical threshold of alcohol toxicity could be estimated because (1) the risk for total abstainers was significantly lower than the risk for people drinking only a low quantity of alcohol (about 1–20 g/day), and (2) even people with extremely high consumption of alcohol may not develop the disease. Besides the quantity of alcohol intake, the duration of alcohol abuse also seems to be important for the development of CP. In females, the disease becomes clinically apparent after a mean of 10–13 years of alcohol consumption and in males after 17 and 18 years [18, 19]. On the other hand, the type of alcoholic beverage or the system of alcohol consumption is not a major factor in the pathogenesis of CP [20]. The mechanism by which alcohol induces CP remains, however, unsettled. Doubtless with regard to morbidity and mortality, the effect of alcohol on the pancreas differs from its effect on the liver. Death rate from alcoholic liver disease in Switzerland is with 11.8 per 100,000 inhabitants per year remarkably higher compared to 0.4 per 100,000 inhabitants per year for alcoholic CP [21, 22]. Interestingly, alcoholic liver cirrhosis is associated with CP in only 2–10% [9, 20, 23, 24]. In an excellent review, Malagelada [25] discussed three major hypotheses of the pathogenesis of alcoholic pancreatitis: (1) toxic effects of alcohol on pancreatic acinar cells; (2) 'plugging' of pancreatic ductules by proteinaceous inhibiting calcium carbonate crystal formation, and (3) reflux of bilioduodenal juice into the pancreatic duct.

The ductal plug hypothesis is now generally accepted as the basic mechanism of alcoholic CP. The key elements are (1) a disturbed regulation of pancreatic secretion by alcohol; (2) an increased secretion of protein, and (3) changes in the composition of pancreatic juice favouring precipitation of protein on formation of protein-calcium complexes.

The interaction of these three variables is complex leading to intraductal formation of protein plugs with and without calcification, resulting in obstruction, inflammation and degeneration of acinar tissue.

Molecular biological analysis of pancreatic protein secretion in patients with chronic calcifying pancreatitis showed that the decrease of a special low-molecular-weight protein, the so-called pancreatic stone protein, is responsible for plug and stone formation in the supersaturated pancreatic juice [26, 27]. This protein, which was originally isolated from the organic matrix of pancreatic stones has also identified in normal pancreatic juice [28] and zymogen granules of pancreatic acinar cells [29]. It has a relatively strong affinity for calcium, thus inhibiting calcium carbonate crystal formation.

Malnutrition

In many developing countries another entity of CP is prevalent. This disease, which is characterized by pancreatic calculi and diabetes mellitus, occurs almost exclusively among children and young nonalcoholic adults in the poorest segments of these societies. This form has been described for many parts of India (with the highest incidence in the state of Kerala) [30], Indonesia [31] and Africa [32]. This so-called tropical pancreatitis (TP) appears to consist of a heterogenous group of diseases with minor histological differences from alcoholic pancreatitis [33]. The

Table 2. Incidence of chronic pancreatitis

Periods	Number of cases	Incidence (per 10^5)	Region	Etiology alcohol, %
1958–1962 [2]	15	0.15	Zurich	53
1963–1972 [14]	102	1.02	Zurich	64
1972–1982 [9]	164	1.64	Zurich	78
1970–1974 [13]	50	6.9	Copenhagen	42
1975–1979 [13]	76	10.0	Copenhagen	71

etiology of TP still remains enigmatic. One of the causes attributed to CP in the tropics was protein malnutrition [32, 34]. However, by detailed dietary enquiry in TP patients and controls no differences in protein or caloric intake could be shown [35] in contrast to fat intake which was low in both groups. Whether the low fat intake of the Kerala population could predispose them to TP as postulated in the case of alcoholic pancreatitis is conjectural [36]. Since the geographic distribution of tropical CP almost conincides in areas where cassava (tapioca) production and consumption is high as in Nigeria, Uganda and Kerala, cassava was thought to be a causative factor in TP. The hydrocyanic acid content of cassava is alleged to cause a toxic effect on the pancreas [37, 38]. It might also deprive the gland of essential amino acids, so vital to its integrity by divesting them of hydrocyanic acid detoxification. At present there is no distinct clinical or experimental evidence that cassava causes TP, but its consumption could have an additive role. The exact etiology of TP remains uncertain.

Idiopathic Chronic Pancreatitis

This form is difficult to define because no threshold level of alcohol toxicity exists and the influence of nutritional factors is often difficult to exclude. Some studies published recently point to the role of the sphincter of Oddi in idiopathic CP. Okazaki et al. [39] showed that in alcoholic and idiopathic CP the basal pressure of the sphincter of Oddi correlates with pancreatic duct pressure. Another allusion for the importance of this pathophysiological mechanism was published by Neoptolemos et al. [40] who found in careful follow-up studies of patients labelled as idiopathic CP, including duodenal bile crystal analysis, evidence of biliary tract stone formation in this group of patients. Furthermore, in a small study of 58 patients with CP who had pancreaticoduodenectomy, 14% were identified with obstructive pancreatopathy due to different causes like duodenal wall cysts, intraductal carcinoma, ectopic pancreatic tissue and neuroendocrine tumors around the papilla [41]. Similar case reports [42, 43] support the hypothesis that the structural and functional integrity of the sphincter of Oddi plays an important role in the etiology of idiopathic CP.

Taking the age of the patients as a basis, idiopathic CP can be divided into juvenile and senile pancreatitis. In Ammann's group of patients with idiopathic CP, 13 had a mean age of 21 years at onset of the disease. All patients suffered from recurrent attacks of acute pancreatitis which in 7 started before the age of 25 years [44]. In none of them was evidence of heredity found. Forty-five of the patients studied were distinctly older at time of diagnosis with 71% beyond the age of 60 years [45]. Two thirds had primary painless CP, the first clinical symptom being mainly weight loss, diarrhea (n = 17) and/or diabetes (n = 8). Men are preferentially affected by both forms. Calcifications on plain X-rays are a typical finding. Possibly, there is a connection between stones in the pancreatic duct in the aged [46] and idiopathic 'senile' pancreatitis [47].

Hereditary Pancreatitis

The initial description of hereditary chronic pancreatitis was given by Comfort et al. [48] in 1952. Ten years later, this form was described in five kindreds who developed recurrent attacks of abdominal pain beginning in early childhood, which affected 21 of 38 patients studied [49]. Transmission follows an autosomal-dominant trait with variable penetrance [50]. In India, a family incidence of 8% was reported in patients with nonalcoholic TP [51].

Congenital Abnormalities

The question whether pancreas divisum predisposes for CP is still open to debate. Sahel et al. [52] showed that pancreas divisum predisposes to acute, but not to chronic pancreatitis [52]. Also, Mitchell et al. [53] were unable to demonstrate a relationship between CP and this congenital abnormality. On the other hand, Cotton [54, 55] remains firmly convinced that there is an etiological association, albeit in a small group of patients. This opinion is supported by the data of Tulassay and Papp [56] who observed a significantly elevated prevalence of pancreatitis in patients with pancreas divisum; unfortunately, no distinction was made between acute and chronic pancreatitis. It is possible that pancreas divisum alone is irrelevant; however, there may be a group of patients in whom abnormalities of the accessory papilla render this abnormality important. Perhaps better diagnostic possibilities like manometry of the accessory sphincter or ultrasound of the dorsal duct system which allows the diagnosis of functional and significant organic stenosis in the minor papilla may answer the question and may help select those patients suitable for surgical or endoscopic treatment.

Metabolic Abnormalities

Hypercalcemia due to hyperparathyroidism may theoretically progress from acute reversible pancreatitis to irreversible organ damage of CP [57–59]. A study by Hirskovic et al. [57] estimated a 3.3% incidence of CP in 450 patients operated because of hyperparathyroidism. CP develops independently of the type of hyperparathyroidism (benign, malignant or hereditary).

Hyperlipidemia types I, IV and V are well-recognized causes of acute pancreatitis but, as for hyperparathyroidism, their role in chronic and calcifying disease rests on less firm ground [60].

Rare Causes

Blunt abdominal trauma may cause pancreatic duct injury leading to incomplete healing or stenosis of the pancreatic duct. These obstructive changes in the duct may promote CP.

Two cases of chronic calcifying pancreatitis were observed after *renal transplantation* [61]. However, other factors like drug therapy may be involved in this situation.

Gallstone disease as the cause of CP was initially suspected at the Mayo Clinic [62]. However, this relationship is unlikely because gallstone disease is present only in a very small percentage of patients with CP. On the other hand, secondary damage to the biliary system is not an uncommon phenomenon affecting 2–55% with this disease [2–13].

While acute pancreatitis is a well-known complication of *drug therapy*, the relationship between drugs and CP is much less evident. In 1981, Ammann et al. [63] described an association between analgetica abuse and CP. This observation was confirmed in a further analysis of a larger group of patients [64]. The association between CP complicated by pseudocyst formation and treatment with prednisone and thiazide was subject to another case report [65].

Natural History of Chronic Pancreatitis

The analysis of the natural history of CP is based on four main factors, namely (1) etiology; (2) clinical pattern and therapy (surgery); (3) morphology, and (4) pancreatic exocrine function. All these factors have to be monitored and interrelated particularly in regard to the time axis from onset to advanced stages of the disease. In the clinical picture and long-term course, nonalcoholic CP differs in certain essential respects from alcoholic CP.

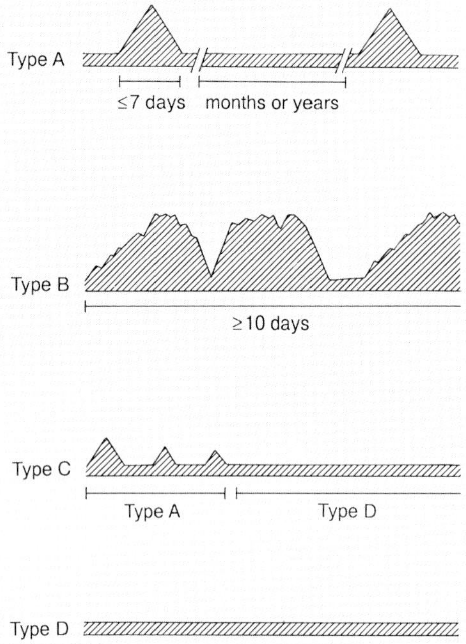

Fig. 1. Typical pain profile of CP. Type A = Recurrent attacks with pain-free intervals; type B = persisting pain; type C = painless CP following recurrent attacks of acute pancreatitis; type D = primary painless CP.

Table 3. Clinical course of chronic pancreatitis

1	Early stage Recurrent attacks of acute pancratitis
2	Late Stage Exocrine and/or exocrine pancreatic insufficiency plus painlessness
3	Complicated disease Persisting pain (or recurrent short-lasting attacks of pain) plus elevated serum levels of pancreatic enzymes and/or local complications

Alcoholic Chronic Pancreatitis (AICP)

Based on the results of a prospective longitudinal study of 163 patients with chronic alcoholic pancreatitis, Ammann et al. [9] showed that clinical picture, morphology and function had typical correlative changes.

Three typical models of disease course can be subdivided from the clinico-biologic and morphologic viewpoint (table 3): (1) an early stage; (2) the late stage, and (3) the complicated disease, CP with local complications (chiefly pseudocysts and duct obstruction).

The basic clinical picture of CP in the early stage consists of recurrent attacks of acute pancreatitis during the first 5 years [66]. In the late stage there is a close relationship between pain attacks and pancreatic function as well as the duration of the disease [9, 67, 68]. Figure 1 shows a typical profile of pain in CP. In the early stages of CP acute recurrent episodic pain attacks are clinically and biochemically indistinguishable from acute pancreatitis (fig. 1, type A). They may probably be due to episodes of acinar inflammation. As a rule, pain attacks are of short duration lasting less than 7 days with pain-free intervals of months or years. In our patients, hospitalizations for severe pain episodes within the first 5 years from onset were necessary 0–1 times in 51%, 2–3 times in 37% and 4 times or more in 12% of patients. It is well established that alcohol withdrawal is the only causal therapy to prevent recurrences. In patients with continuing alcohol abuse pain attacks will be less severe and less common with progression of duration of the disease. This is related to a progressive destruction of acinar tissue. In the late stage when most of the glandular tissue is destroyed there is a complete pain relief which is paralleled by a significant decrease in exocrine pandreatic function (fig. 1, type C) because the substrate for acinar inflammation is lost. Long-lasting pain relief (more than 2 years without pain) occurred in

Table 4. Indications and surgical procedures in 120 patients

Diagnosis	Indications		Technique		
	cysts	pain (no cysts)	drainage procedure[1]	PJ	resection[2]
AICP	76	23	33	38	28
NAICP	12	9	8	9	4
Σ	88	32	41	47	32

PJ = Pancreatico-jejunostomy.
1 Cyst drainage, either by castojejunostomy or external drainage.
2 Mainly left pancreatectomy (40–60%).

131 of 159 patients with alcoholic CP (82.4%). The mean duration of pain from the first to the last episode in 133 patients who got lasting pain relief (for 2 years or longer) was 4.5 ± 2.9 (0.5–14) years. It occurred at a similar rate for the both operated and the unoperated (n = 86) groups.

In the late stage of uncomplicated CP, the disease is dominated by pancreatic insufficiency, i.e. diabetes or steatorrhea without pain. That means uncomplicated CP (fig. 1, type A) proceeds in the late stage to painless CP (fig. 1, type C).

The third typical disease pattern is complicated CP, characterized by persistent pain (or recurrences at short intervals) (fig. 1, type B). This clinical pain pattern which is accompanied by elevation of pancreatic serum enzymes is nearly exclusively caused by the development of local complications, like pseudocysts, extrahepatic cholestasis or pancreatic obstruction [9]. Sometimes pain is associated with marked weight loss mimicking pancreatic cancer. These local complications can easily be diagnosed by ultrasound, computer tomography or ERCP and cured by surgery (usually using drainage procedures). As shown in table 4, 120 out of 287 patients with CP studied regularly over the last 25 years underwent pancreatic surgery [9, 69]. Prompt postoperative pain relief after drainage of the pancreatic pseudocysts was observed in 26 of 51 patients (51%). However, episodic pain relapses postoperatively are quite common, particularly in the early stages of the disease and if alcohol abuse is continued. Of the 25 patients with postoperative pain relapses 19 (37%) got lasting pain relief for an average of only 2.9 years after surgery. These data show that complicated CP with lasting pain syndrome can be reconverted by surgical erradication of local complications into uncomplicated CP.

Nonalcoholic Chronic Pancreatitis (NAICP)

A comparison of the natural history of the disease in 205 patients with alcohol-induced pancreatitis with 82 patients in whom alcohol could not be incriminated as a cause shows remarkable similarities as well as differences [9, 70]. Both groups showed progressive exocrine insufficiency and, thus, the ultimate incidence of steatorrhea (AICP 48%; NAICP 52%), calcification (AICP 85%; NAICP 77%) and death (AICP 41%; NAICP 77%), respectively, was nearly the same in both groups. Another similarity between the two was male predominance suggesting a genetic and possibly even hormonal predilection among men. In the clinical picture and long-term course NAICP differs in certain essential respects from AICP. Prgression of exocrine insufficiency from the time of diagnosis in NAICP is much slower than in AICP. Diabetes was less common in NAICP than in AICP at the 6-year follow-up time. Whether this slower progression to exocrine insufficiency had a morphologic counterpart or simply reflects the more rapid progression in those patients with continuous alcohol intake is still a matter of debate [71, 72]. The most striking difference between the two groups was the remarkably higher incidence of painless disease in NAICP (54%) as compared to AICP (5%) (fig. 1, type D). Although pain relief was naturally associated with progressive and marked exocrine insufficiency (especially in AICP), yet in 8 of 27 patients with NAICP pancreatic exocrine function was persistently normal for more than 6 years after the onset of lasting pain relief.

References

1 Comfort MW, Gambill EE, Baggenstoss AH: Chronic relapsing pancreatitis, an analysis of twenty-nine cases without associated disease of the biliary or gastrointestinal tract. Gastroenterology 1946;6:239–285, 376–408.

2 Hämmerli UP, Hefti MI, Schmid M: Chronic pancreatitis in Zurich, 1958 through 1962. Bibl Gastroenterol 1965;7:58–63.

3 White TT, Murat J, Morgan A: Pancreatitis. Review of 733 cases of pancreatitis from the Seattle hospitals. Northwest Med 1968;67:374–377.

4 Creutzfeldt W, Fehr H, Schmidt H: Verlaufsbeobachtungen und diagnostische Verfahren bei der chronisch rezidivierenden und chronischen Pankreatitis. Schweiz Med Wochenschr 1970;100:1180–1189.

5 Gastard J, Jouband F, Farbos T, et al: Etiology and course of primary chronic pancreatitis in Western France. Digestion 1973;9:416–428.

6 Gullo I, Costa PL, Labo G: Chronic pancreatitis in Italy. Aetiological, clinical and histological observations based on 253 cases. Rendiconti Gastroenterol 1977;9:97–102.

7 White TT, Slavotinek AH: Results of surgical treatment of chronic pancreatitis. Ann Surg 1979;189:217–224.

8 Aldrete JS, Jimenez H, Halpern NB: Evaluation and treatment of acute and chronic pancreatitis. A review of 380 cases. Ann Surg 1980;191:664–671.

9 Ammann RW, Akovbiantz A, Largiadér F, Schueler G: Course and outcome of chronic pancreatitis. Gastroenterology 1984;86:820–828.

10 Goebell H, Hotz J, Hoffmeister H: Hypercaloric nutrition as an aetiological factor in chronic pancreatitis. Z Gastroenterol 1980;18:94–97.

11 Copenhagen Pancreatitis Study: An interim report from a prospective epidemiological multicenter study. Scand J Gastroenterol 1981;17:247.

12 Kondo T, Hayakawa T, Noda A, et al: Follow up study of chronic pancreatitis. Gastroenterol Jpn 1981;16:46–53.

13 Andersen BN, Pedersen NT, Scheel J, Worning H: Incidence of alcoholic chronic pancreatitis in Copenhagen. Scand J Gastroenterol 1982;17:247–252.

14 Ammann RW, Hammer B, Fumagalli I: Chronic pancreatitis in Zurich, 1963–1972. Digestion 1973;9:404–415.

15 Vantini I, Gavallini G, Angelini G, et al: Nutritional aspects of chronic pancreatitis in Verona, Italy. Rendiconti Gastroenterol 1977;9:13–16.

16 Voirol M, Infante F, Brahime-Reteno O, et al: Consommation d'alcool, de tabac et de nutriments dans les affections pancréatiques. Schweiz Med Wochenschr 1980;110:854–855.

17 Sarles H, Sarles JC, Camatte R, Muratore R, Gaini M, Guien C, Pastor J, Leroy F: Observations on 205 confirmed cases of acute pancreatitis, recurring pancreatitis and chronic pancreatitis. Gut 1965;6:545–559.

18 Durbec JP, Sarles H: Multicenter survey of the etiology of pancreatic diseases. Relationship between the relative risk of developing chronic pancreatitis and alcohol, protein and lipid consumption. Digestion 1978;18:337–350.

19 Pitchumoni CS, Sonnenshein M, Candido FM, et al: Nutrition in the pathogenesis of alcoholic pancreatitis. Am J Clin Nutr 1980;33:631–638.

20 Sarles H, Cros RG, Bidart JM: An international group for study of pancreatic diseases: A multicenter inquiry into the etiology of pancreatic diseases. Digestion 1979;19:110–125.

21 Muster E: Zahlen und Fakten zu Alkohol- und Drogenproblemen 1983/84. Lausanne, Verlag SFA, Schweizerische Fachstelle für Alkoholprobleme, 1983.
22 Ammann RW: Epidemiology and etiology of chronic pancreatitis in Zurich; in Sato T, Yamaudi H (eds): Pancreatitis. Tokyo, University of Tokyo Press, 1985.
23 Dürr HK: Alkoholschädigung des Pankreas. Internist (Berlin) 1978; 19:123–130.
24 Singer MV, Sarles H, Goebell H: Chronische Pankreatitis; in Demling L (ed): Klinische Gastroenterologie, ed 2, vol 2. Stuttgart, Thieme, 1984, pp 445–477.
25 Malagelada JR: The pathophysiology of alcoholic pancreatitis. Pancreas 1986;1:270–278.
26 Guy O, Robles-Diaz G, Adrich Z, Sahel J, Sarles H: Protein content of precipitates present in pancreatic juice of alcoholic subjects and patients with chronic calcifying pancreatitis. Gastroenterology 1983;84: 102–107.
27 De Caro A, Multigner L, Lafont H, Lombardo D, Sarles H: The molecular characteristics of a human pancreatic acidic phosphoprotein that inhibits calcium carbonate crystal growth. Biochem J 1984;222:669–677.
28 De Caro A, Lohse J, Sarles H: Characterisation of a protein isolated from pancreatic calculi of men suffering from chronic calcifying pancreatitis. Biochem Biophys Res Commun 1979;87:1176–1182.
29 Lechene de la Porte P, De Caro A, Amonvic M, Sarles H: Localisation immunocytochimique de la protéine majoritaire des calculs pancréatiques humains. Nouvelle Presse Méd 1981;10:3851.
30 Kanshik SP, Kochhar P, Metha SK: Spectrum of chronic pancreatitis at Chandigarth. Tiruchirapalli, Chronic pancreatitis in India. St. Joseph's Press, 1987.
31 Zuidema PJ: Cirrhosis and disseminated calcification of the pancreas in patients with malnutrition. Trop Geogr Med 1959;11:70–74.
32 Shaper AG: Aetiology of chronic pancreatic fibrosis with calcification seen in Uganda. Br Med J 1964;i: 1607–1609.
33 Balaraman NM, Latha P: Pancreas in chronic calcific pancreatitis. Chronic pancreatitis in India. St. Joseph's Press, 1987, pp 115–120.
34 Retnaike VT, Rajassuria K: Pancreatic calcification related to protein malnutrition. Trop Geogr Med 1963;15:1–4.
35 Balakrishnan V: In Bernades P, Hugier M (eds): Pancreatic tropicale. Maladies du pancréas exocrine. Paris, Doin, 1987.
36 Balakrishnan B, Sauniere JF, Hariharan M, et al: Diet, pancreatic function and chronic pancreatitis in South India and in France. Pancreas 1988;3:30–35.
37 McMillan DE, GeeVarghese PJ: Dietary cyanide and tropical malnutrition diabetes. Diabetes Care 1979;2: 202–208.
38 Pitchumoni CS: Special problems of tropical pancreatitis. Clin Gastroenterol 1984;13:941–959.
39 Okazaki K, Yamamoto Y, Nishimori I, Nishioka T, Kagiyama S, Tamura S, Sakamoto Y, Nakazawa Y, Morita M, Yamamoto I: Motility of the sphincter of Oddi and pancreatic main ductal pressure in patients with alcoholic, gallstone-associated, and idiopathic chronic pancreatitis. Am J Gastroenterol 1988;83:820–826.
40 Neoptolemos JP, Davidson BR, Winder AF, Valance D: Role of duodenal bile crystal analysis in the investigation of 'idiopathic' pancreatitis. Br J Surg 1988;75:450–453.
41 Lowes JR, Rode J, Lees WR, Russel RCG, Cotton PB: Obstructive pancreatitis: Unusual causes of chronic pancreatitis. Br J Surg 1988;75: 1129–1132.
42 Gettenberg G, Zimbalist E, Marini D: Chronic pancreatitis and pseudocyst formation secondary to carcinoid tumor of the pancreas. Gastroenterology 1988;94:1222–1224.
43 Malhotra R, Evans R, Bhawan J, Kanzaria P, Silva W: A malignant gastric leiomyoblastoma presenting as an infected pseudocyst of the pancreas. Am J Gastroenterol 1988;83: 452–456.
44 Ammann RW: Die idiopathisch «juvenile» chronische Pankreatitis. Dtsch Med Wochenschr 1976;101: 1789–1794.
45 Ammann RW, Sulser H: Die «senile» chronische Pankreatitis – eine neue nosologische Einheit? Schweiz Med Wochenschr 1976;106:429–437.
46 Nagai H, Ohtsbo K: Pancreatic lithiasis in the aged. Gastroenterology 1984;86:331–338.
47 Ammann RW: Idiopathic 'senile' chronic pancreatitis and pancreatic lithiasis in the aged. Gastroenterology 1984;87:153.
48 Comfort WM, Steinberg AG: Pedigree of a family with hereditary chronic relapsing pancreatitis. Gastroenterology 1952;21:54–63.
49 Gross J, Gambill EE, Ulrich JA: Hereditary pancreatitis. Description of fifth kindred an summary of clinical features. Am J Med 1962;33:358–362.
50 Stafford RJ, Grand RJ: Hereditary disease of the exocrine pancreas. Clin Gastroenterol 1982;11:141–170.
51 GeeVarghese PJ, Pitchumoni CS: Pancreatic diabetes in Kerala. Based on a clinico-pathological study of 325 diabetic patient with pancreatic calculi. Proc World Congr Diabetes in the Tropics, Bombay.
52 Sahel J, Cros RC, Bourri J, Sarles H: Clinicopathological conditions associated with pancreas divisum. Digestion 1982;23:1–8.
53 Mitchell CJ, Lintott DJ, Ruddell WSJ, et al: Clinical relevance of an unfused pancreatic duct system. Gut 1979;20:1066–1071.
54 Cotton PB: Congenital anomaly of pancreas divisum as a cause of obstructive pain and pancreatitis. Gut 1980;21:105–114.
55 Cotton PB: Pancreas divisum. Pancreas 1988;3:245–247.
56 Tulassay Z, Papp J: New clinical aspects of pancreas divisum. Gastrointest Endsocopy 1980;26:143–146.
57 Hirskovic T, Keating FR, Gross IB: Coexistent pancreatitis and hyperparathyreoidism. Observations in 15 cases. Gastroenterology 1967;52: 1093.
58 Creutzfeldt W, Schmidt H: Pankreatitis beim primären Hyperparathyreoidismus und Calciphylaxie. Tijdscrift Gastroenterol 1965;8: 385–392.

59 Goebell H, Horn HD, Bode C, Grossmann HH: Primärer Hyperparathyreoidismus und exokrine Pankreasfunktion. Störungen der Enzym- und Elektrolytsekretion im Duodenalsaft beim Sekretin-Pankreozymintest. Klin Wochenschr 1970;48:810–819.
60 Farmer RG, Winkelmann EI, Brown HB, Lewis LA: Hyperlipoproteinemia and pancreatitis. Am J Med 1973;54:161–165.
61 Corrodi P, Knoblauch M, Binswanger V, Schölzel E, Largiadér F: Pancreatitis after renal transplantation. Gut 1975;16:285–289.
62 Gambill EE, Comfort MW: Chronic relapsing pancreatitis: An analysis of 27 cases associated with disease of the biliary tract. Gastroenterology 1948;11:1–33.
63 Ammann RW, Bühler H, Tuma J, Schneider J, Siebenmann R, Satz N: Chronic and relapsing acute pancreatitis associated with chronic renal insufficiency and analgesic (phenacetin) abuse. Gastroenterol Clin Biol 1981;5:509–514.
64 Hangartner P, Bühler H, Münch R, Zaruba K, Stamm B, Ammann RW: Chronische Pankreatitis als wahrscheinliche Folge eines Analgetikaabusus. Schweiz Med Wochenschr 1987;117:638–642.
65 Weaver GA, Bordley J, Guiney WB, D'Accurzio A: Chronic pancreatitis with cyst formation after prednisone and thiazide treatment. Am J Gastroentérol 1982;77:164–168.
66 Bernades P, Belghiti J, Athouel M, Mallardo N, Breil P, Fekete F: Histoire naturelle de la pancréatite chronique. Etude de 120 cas. Gastroenterol Clin Biol 1983;7:8–13.
67 Ammann RW: Diagnose und Therapie der alkoholischen chronischen Pankreatitis. Eine Standortbestimmung. Schweiz Med Wochenschr 1985;115(suppl 19):42–51.
68 Ammann RW: Alcohol- and nonalcohol-induced pancreatitis: Clinical aspects; in Burns G, Bank S (eds): Disorders of the Pancreas. Controversies in Diagnosis and Management. New York, MacMillan, 1989.
69 Ammann RW: Klinik, Spontanverlauf und Therapie der chronischen Pankreatitis. Schweiz Med Wochenschr 1983;119:696–706.
70 Ammann RW, Buehler H, Muench R, Freiburghaus A, Siegenthaler W: Differences in the natural history of idiopathic (non-alcoholic) and alcoholic chronic pancreatitis. Pancreas 1987;3:368–377.
71 Nagata A, Homma T, Tamai K, et al: A study of chronic pancreatitis by serial endoscopic pancreatography. Gastroenterology 1981;81:884–891.
72 Girdwood AH, Gilinsky NH, Hatfield HRN, et al: Duplicate pancreatic function testing in chronic pancreatitis. Abstr First Int Meet Pancreatology, Lisboa, 1984, pp 1–64.

Dig Dis 1992;10:345–353

H.G. Gooszen

Department of Surgery,
University Hospital, Leiden,
The Netherlands

Surgical Treatment of Painful Chronic Pancreatitis: An Unresolved Problem?

Key Words
Chronic pancreatitis
Early surgery
Operative strategy

Abstract
Relief of pain in chronic pancreatitis is the major problem warranting surgical treatment in this disease. The mechanism of pain is largely unknown and several types of operation have been devised for treatment. Side-to-side pancreaticojejunostomy (Partington-Rochelle) and pancreaticoduodenectomy according to Whipple have stood the test of time. Recently, new surgical options have been explored like the operation according to Beger, segmental autotransplantation, and duodenum-preserving total pancreatectomy. Because of the reluctance to refer this type patient for surgery, treatment with analgesic drugs is continued for quite some time and once analgesia addiction has developed clinical judgement in these patients is severely hampered. Surgery can be performed with 70–80% success and with limited morbidity as well as low mortality. For these reasons surgery should be discussed early in the disease if pain becomes a major problem. If these patients are operated prior to analgesia addiction, maybe the long-term prognosis will improve. The diagnostic and surgical approach will be discussed in detail with a plea for considering surgery early in the course of disease.

Introduction

Chronic pancreatitis is a disease initiated as a focal or as a diffuse inflammatory process. The incidence of the disease in the Western world is slowly rising from below 1 to 10 per 100,000 inhabitants per year [1]. The disease is usually caused by alcohol overindulgence and the exact mechanism of pancreatic tissue destruction is not fully understood. In about 30% of patients, the disease is of idiopathic origin. The damage to the pancreas is

H.G. Gooszen, MD
Department of Surgery, Building 43
University Hospital Leiden
PO Box 9600
NL-2300 RC Leiden (The Netherlands)

© 1992
S. Karger AG, Basel
0257–2753/92/
0106–0345$2.75/0

progressive irrespective of the type of treatment. Abstinence of alcohol is mandatory but will not stop progression of the morphological changes in the majority of patients. Although some data are currently presented that effective surgery can stop progression of tissue damage [2], one should not expect improvement of pancreatic morphology and function after surgery for this condition. Surgery in complicated chronic pancreatitis is meant for palliation of a benign disease with a course usually leading to progressive loss of function, diabetes mellitus and exocrine insufficiency. The disease decreases life expectancy and after a mean disease duration of 10 years only 50% of the patients are still alive [3]. There is no effect of surgical treatment on survival. Histologically, the disease is characterized by focal, segmental or diffuse sclerosis with progressive loss of acinar and endocrine tissue, with or without (segmental) dilatation of the pancreatic ductal system.

The clinical presentation of chronic pancreatitis shows large variations. The disease can present as painful chronic pancreatitis of a recurrent or persistent type. Chronic pancreatitis can be primarily painless or can 'burn out' to secondary painless disease after a period of usually intermittent episodes of pain. Primary painless pancreatitis is rare (5%) if the disease is caused by alcohol, but much more frequent (50%) if alcohol can be excluded as the cause of chronic pancreatitis.

The disease can run an uncomplicated course, but there is the group of patients with intractable persistent pain that can lead to surgical intervention and, independent of the presence of pain, complications like pseudocyst formation, obstructive jaundice, duodenal obstruction and portal hypertension can occur at any stage of the disease process. Obstructive jaundice or other signs and complications of a pseudocyst can be the first presentation of the disease and do not need to be preceded by attacks of upper abdominal pain. Interpretation of the severity of pain represents a major problem in patients with chronic pancreatitis, especially if induced by alcohol overindulgence. The mechanism of pain in chronic pancreatitis is still largely obscure and two different mechanisms have been proposed; the dilatation type of pain and the perineural inflammation-induced type of pain [4].

The dilatation type of pain can explain the chronic pain in patients with pancreatic pseudocyst and in those with gross ductal dilatation. Perineural inflammation probably plays a key role in focal and in diffuse pancreatitis with or without ductal dilatation.

The course and spontaneous evolution of pain in the individual patient is the major concern if surgical intervention is considered.

Based on his large experience in the observation and treatment of patients with chronic pancreatitis, Ammann has distinguished three types of pancreatic pain based on the clinical course in a large group of patients. Type A pain is the type of pain observed in patients with recurrent attacks of pain and uncomplicated pancreatitis. Intervals between the attacks may be months or years. Type B pain is observed in patients with obstructive disease, at a ductular level, and in those with pseudocyst, pancreatic cancer or analgesic drug abuse.

In patients with secondary painless pancreatitis, type A pain progresses into the type C subgroup. This course of the disease is referred to as the 'burning out' process. He advises medical treatment for types A and C and surgery for the type B clinical course [5]. To use this classification in clinical practice implies the need for observation for sometimes over a year to decide upon surgical intervention, or continuation of a conservative approach.

Indications for Surgical Relief of Pain

If exocrine substitution therapy has failed to relieve severe pain, and analgesic drugs like paracetamol, diclofenac and the like are ineffective, surgical treatment should be discussed. Mortality, even of major operations, should be low and a proper selection of the type of operation needed can only be assessed after thorough clinical and radiological examination. Surgical intervention is never acute so patients can go through a detailed work-up including consultation with a social worker, psychologist or psychiatrist. The patient should be fully aware of the extent and consequences of the operation and the fact that surgery can in no way beneficially influence the disease. They should also be able to cope with a life-style with dietary restrictions, insulin administration and exocrine substitution, especially if they are about to undergo major ablative surgery.

A pancreatic pseudocyst can induce severe pain and can only be excluded as the cause if percutaneous puncture does not lead to pain relief. Common bile duct obstruction with or without jaundice can be observed in patients with painful chronic pancreatitis.

Jaundice can occur in the course of chronic pancreatitis and can be caused by a pseudocyst in the head of the pancreas, by progressive fibrosis in the pancreatic head as part of progressive destruction with subsequent scar formation of pancreatic tissue (fig. 1) or by edema during an exacerbation of chronic pancreatitis.

If partial or subtotal common bile duct obstruction is accompanied by chronic pancreatic pain, biliary bypass is sufficient to decompress the biliary system, but decompression should not be expected to contribute to the relief of pain. Bile duct stenosis as such, however, is not a well-known cause of chronic pain and a coexisting pseudocyst in the head of the pancreas or a focal lesion with fibrosis and secondary bile duct compression should be held responsible.

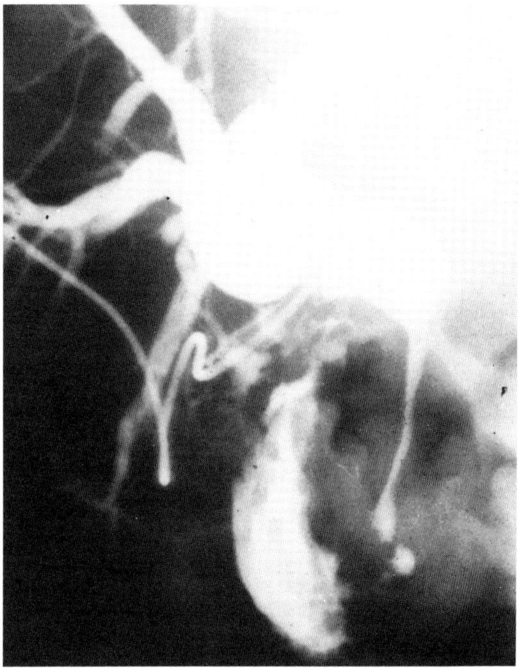

Fig. 1. Biliary tract stricture secondary to chronic pancreatitis and fibrosis in the head of the pancreas.

Contraindications for Surgery

Portal hypertension, persistent alcoholism and analgesic drug addiction represent relative contraindications to surgery especially if pancreatic pain is the reason for considering surgical treatment.

Portal hypertension as a result of alcohol liver disease can coexist with alcohol-induced chronic pancreatitis and represents an increased risk for intraoperative blood loss and postoperative complications. The condition should be differentiated from segmental por-

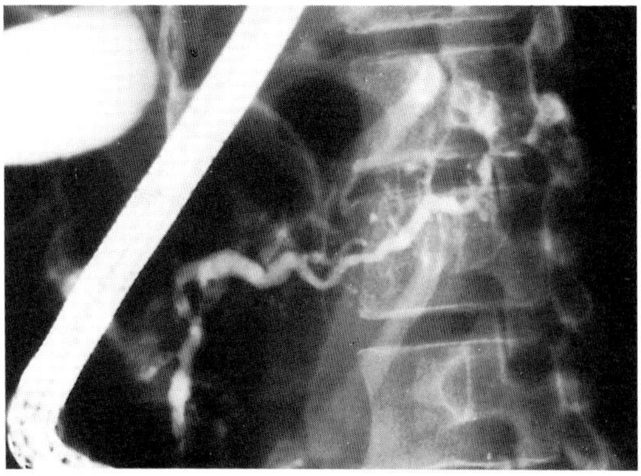

Fig. 2. Diffuse disease in a patient with alcohol-induced chronic pancreatitis.

tal hypertension secondary to splenic vein thrombosis. This is not a major risk factor and can be dealt with by splenectomy or distal splenic artery ligation if the patient has not bled from fundal varices. If the patient is about to undergo pancreaticojejunostomy or resection of the pancreatic head, splenectomy or splenic artery ligation should preferably be performed as the first step of the operation.

Persistent alcoholism is a relative contraindication to surgery since it compromises the outcome of surgical treatment and it increases morbidity not so much by the operation itself but by the fact that these patients cannot comply with the implications of major surgery like endocrine and exocrine substition. Essentially, the same holds for addiction to analgesic drugs.

Preoperative Work-Up

With the introduction of ultrasound, CT scanning and ERCP, confirmation of the diagnosis of chronic pancreatitis is no longer a major problem. The preoperative work-up is dictated by the complication of the disease that represents the indication for surgery.

In case of otherwise *intractable pain*, detailed information about persistent alcohol abuse and about analgesic drug addiction is the mainstay of the preoperative work-up. Ultrasonography is particularly useful in showing a pancreatic pseudocyst. CT scanning can give more-detailed information on the damage done to the pancreatic parenchyma, the relation of the inflammatory tissue to the surrounding structures like the duodenum, the spleen, the portal vein and the biliary system. ERCP delineates morphological changes of the common bile duct and the pancreatic duct with its side branches.

The result of the preoperative ERCP, especially the degree of ductal dilatation, dictates the type of operation.

With relevance to the type of operation, ductal changes can be subdivided into three main groups; diffuse disease without significant ductal dilatation (fig. 2), right-sided lesions in the head of the pancreas with gross diffuse ductal dilatation (fig. 3) or without significant (fig. 4) secondary changes in body and tail, and left-sided ductal changes. Additional evaluation of exocrine and endocrine function helps in deciding what definitive operation is selected: 'minor operation in case of minor functional damage and a major resection (total or subtotal pancreatectomy) only in case of gross functional destruction'. Surgery for chronic pancreatitis can nowadays be performed with mortality rates below 3% and effectivity ranging to about 80%. Operation for otherwise intractable pain should only be performed after very careful evaluation of the patients' clinical history, and diagnostic work-up should not be postponed until a previous alcoholic has changed into an analgesia addict with insulin-dependent diabetes mellitus. Effective operations should not be withheld from patients in an

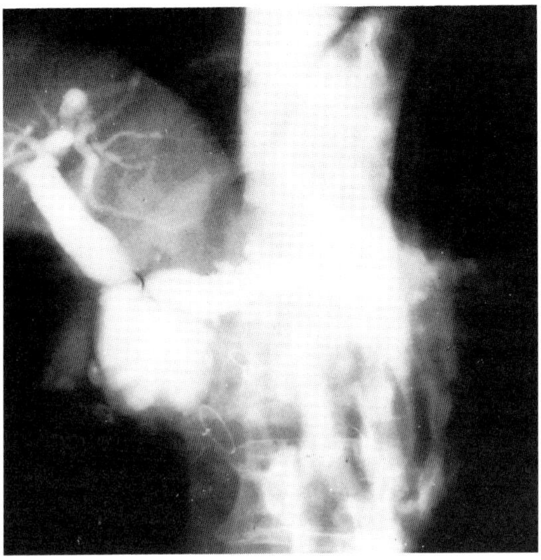

Fig. 3. Dilatation of the common bile duct and pancreatic duct secondary to gross changes in the head of the pancreas. Pseudocyst puncture did not lead to normalisation of diameter of either of the ducts.

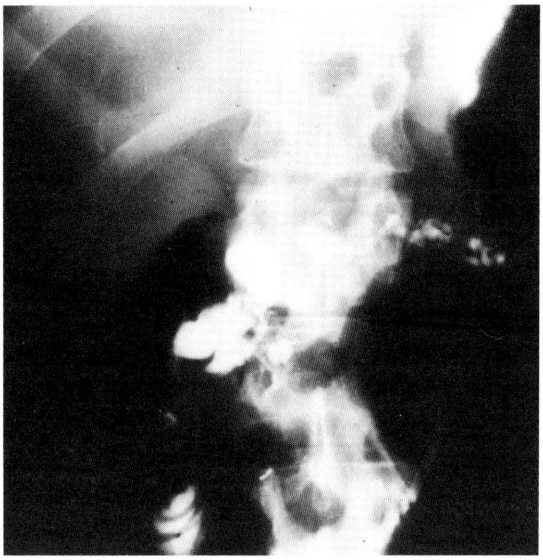

Fig. 4. Chronic pancreatitis with morphological changes mainly in the pancreatic head. Minor changes in pancreatic duct diameter are observed in body and tail.

early stage of the disease based on fatalistic considerations, and therefore ERCP, CT scanning and evaluation of pancreatic function should be performed early in the disease process, with the intent to look for a surgically correctable lesion.

Arteriography of the coeliac axis and superior mesenteric artery can detect abnormal vascularisation of the liver and can be helpful in case of resection of the pancreatic head, but can also be performed for late-phase splenoportography if portal hypertension with portal vein occlusion by alcoholic liver cirrhosis is suspected, or if segmental portal hypertension should be confirmed.

If pancreatic pseudocyst is considered the cause of pain and therefore represents the indication for surgery, many authors, including our group, advocate preoperative ERCP to get information about the relation between the pancreatic duct and the pseudocyst to appreciate what type of operation, internal drainage or partial resection, is to preferred [6]. Others plead that preoperative ERCP is dangerous because of the risk of introducing infection into the pseudocyst, that it is costly and not essential for operative decision making [7]. In case of common bile duct stenosis with or without jaundice, ERCP is essential to learn about the length of the stenotic segment. It is important to choose between hepaticojejunostomy and simple choledochoduodenostomy.

Splenic vein thrombosis can be detected on contrast-enhanced CT scanning, because varicose veins in the fundus of the stomach and along the lesser curvature are visualized. This modality also gives detailed information about pancreatic morphology. Therefore, we prefer CT scanning over arteriography/splenoportography under these circumstances.

Operations for the Relief of Pain

Painful chronic pancreatitis can be divided into three groups based on morphological changes observed on CT scanning and ERCP.

(I) Chronic pancreatitis with the inflammatory mass in the head of the pancreas; (II) diffuse type of chronic pancreatitis with or without dilatation of the main pancreatic duct; (III) left-sided pancreatitis: this subdivision has no connection with those devised by Sarner and Cotton [8] and adapted by Singer and Gyr [9], and only serves as a useful guide to select the appropriate operation for the individual patient.

Inflammatory Mass in the Head of the Pancreas

Cephalic pancreaticoduodenectomy according to Whipple is the standard operation in this subgroup. Pain relief is obtained in 60–100% of patients [10–12]. In the classical design, a distal gastrectomy is part of the procedure. Mortality of the procedure is below 5% in expert series and the early postoperative complication rate should also be low. Distal gastrectomy, however, can lead to dumping, peptic ulceration, alkaline reflux gastritis and malabsorption. Adequate exocrine substitution can be very difficult after partial gastrectomy and as a consequence treatment of diabetes mellitus by insulin administration and diet can dangerously be compromised. To avoid distal gastrectomy, the pylorus-preserving pancreaticoduodenectomy (PPPD) has been developed [13] but the operation has not gained widespread popularity. Delayed gastric emptying is one of the most important drawbacks.

To prevent the disadvantages of Whipple's operation and PPPD, Beger et al. [14] have devised the duodenum-preserving resection (DPR) of the head of the pancreas. With this procedure, pylorus, duodenum, common bile duct and gallbladder are left intact and the head of the pancreas is peeled off from the duodenum after transection of the pancreas at the level of the portal vein. Pain relief and mortality rate are in the same range as after Whipple's procedure.

The operation has a very low complication rate and interferes less with upper gastrointestinal physiology than Whipple's procedure or PPPD. The latter argument constitutes the major advantage of the procedure. It seems that the nutritional status of patients after DPR of the pancreatic head is better and that diabetes and exocrine insufficiency are less of a problem than after Whipple's operation and PPPD.

Comparative studies, however, have not been conducted to prove the impression of Beger and co-workers. There is some experimental evidence showing that release patterns of gastrointestinal hormones and pancreatic hormones largely remain intact after DPR [15]. Inoue et al. [16] have shown that CCK release is decreased after Whipple's procedure, irrespective of the type of reconstruction of the upper gastrointestinal tract. In dogs CCK response is unchanged after DPR, if stimulated by a test meal [15].

Diffuse Disease

If morphological changes are diffuse and no specific, restricted area can be identified, the main pancreatic duct can be of normal size or be dilated over its full length. If the duct diameter is 8 mm or more, the procedure as described by Partington and Rochelle [17] is the operation of choice.

The decision to perform a desobstruction-type operation and not a (partial) resection is based on the assumption that dilatation of the main pancreatic duct indicates high pressure in the ductal system and represents the cause of pancreatic pain. There is, however, no solid evidence for an increase in pressure in the main duct in these patients.

There is an understandable preference for the desobstruction-type operation since no pancreatic tissue is resected and no adverse effect on pancreatic exocrine and endocrine function has to be accounted for.

In 1954, DuVal described the distal end-to-end pancreaticojejunostomy after limited distal resection in this group of patients. Recurrence rates of disabling pain turned out to be as high as over 50% and the operation was largely abandoned. Renewed or persistent stenoses in the pancreatic duct in combination with occlusion of the pancreaticojejunostomy were the suspected causes of recurrent pain. The DuVal operation was replaced by the operation designed by Puestow and Gillesby in 1958. In their design, the pancreatic duct was filletted from the tail downstream to the head of the pancreas. The spleen and part of the pancreatic tail were removed and a roux-en-Y limb was anastomosed to the incised pancreatic duct.

In 1960, Partington and Rochelle [17] improved this technique without introducing conceptual changes. No pancreatic tissue is resected in their design and the spleen can also be left in situ.

This procedure found worldwide acceptance and is indicated in patients with chronic pancreatitis, disabling pain and a dilated pancreatic duct up to at least 8 mm in diameter, with or without the so-called 'chain of lakes' aspect.

Short-term favorable effect on pain in 60–90% of the cases, limited effect on pancreatic function and mortality rates of below 5% justify the wide application of the Partington-Rochelle procedure. Long-term pain relief does not exceed 50%.

If there is diffuse disease without ductal dilatation, total pancreatectomy seems the only rational approach. Although the technique has been improved and duodenectomy can even be prevented [18], the morbidity and mortality of the procedure are still unacceptably high [19]. The operation-induced diabetes with a lacking glucagon counterregulation is prone to deep hypoglycemia and patient death of unknown frequency. Alternatives have been devised and segmental autotransplantation of the pancreatic body and tail to the left iliac fossa has been performed with success [20]. The indication for this elaborative procedure is limited. Attempts to isolate islets from the diseased pancreas followed by islet autotransplantation have failed [21].

Left-Sided Pancreatitis

Left-sided pancreatitis seems limited to the nonalcoholic form of chronic pancreatitis. An intraductal carcinoma of the body of the pancreas has to be ruled out. In these patients, 60% left-sided pancreatectomy, with transection at the level of the portal vein, can lead to pain relief. This procedure has been abandoned in patients with alcoholic-induced pancreatitis.

Pain in Chronic Pancreatitis: An Unresolvable Problem?

Are current results sufficient to adapt a more aggressive strategy to patients with painful chronic pancreatitis?

With improvement in perioperative care, anesthesia and operative technique, major operations for chronic pancreatitis are performed with operative mortality rates below 5% in specialized centers. Operative morbidity has been reduced with better regulation of diabetes mellitus and exocrine substitution has been simplified with the introduction of duodenum-preserving resection of the pancreatic head and duodenum-preserving total pancreatectomy. Improved exocrine substitution in its turn facilitates dietary regulation and regulation of diabetes, since dumping and malabsorption as observed after Whipple's procedure are no longer a major problem. Patients with chronic pancreatitis and invaliding pain (type B pain according to Ammann) should have full-scale evaluation at an early stage. If a lesion is found that can be tackled by a nonresection operation (pseudocyst drainage or pancreaticojejunostomy according to Partington-Rochelle), surgical treatment should be proposed. If a distinct lesion in the head of the pancreas is found, both Whipple's procedure and the duodenum-preserving resection according to Beger offer good results with pain relief in 80% of the patients. Based on our own experience, we prefer the Beger-type resection of the pancreatic head, although we are aware of the fact that no studies are available to compare the Whipple- and Beger-type resections of the pancreatic head. We justify our preference in a limited series on the good nutritional condition of our patients with limited problems in diabetes control.

Patients with recurrent pain after surgery represent a neglected problem. Patients who experience recurrence or persistence of disabling pain after an established procedure should not be withheld the chance for renewed surgical intervention provided they are off alcohol and not addicted to analgesic drugs.

We have successfully converted pancreaticojejunostomies into Beger's type resection, and Beger's type resection into segmental autotransplantation or total pancreatectomy, provided the phase of complete endocrine insufficiency has been reached. It has to be kept in mind that no satisfactory explanation for the origin of pain in chronic pancreatitis is available irrespective of the duct diameter, that surgery does not improve survival, and that it has no proven benefit on pancreatic function.

Results of decompression-type procedures should not be compared in their effectiveness to those of any type of resection, since indications differ basically. Although the problem of surgical approach to painful chronic pancreatitis has not been resolved, there is a better defined place for surgical treatment early in the course of the disease.

References

1 Worning H: Incidence and prevalence of chronic pancreatitis; in Beger HG, Büchler M, Ditschuneit H, Malfertheimer P (eds): Chronic Pancreatitis. Berlin, Springer, 1990, pp 8–14.

2 Nelson WH, Townsend CM Jr, Thompson JC: Operative drainage of the pancreatic duct delays functional impairment in patients with chronic pancreatitis. Ann Surg 1988;208:21–329.

3 Ammann RW, Akovbiantz A, Largiadèr F, Schueler G: Course and outcome of chronic pancreatitis. Gastroenterology 1984;86:820–828.

4 Bockman DE, Büchler M, Malfertheimer P, Beger HG: Analysis of nerves in chronic pancreatitis. Gastroenterology 1988;94:1459–1469.

5 Ammann RW: Natural history of chronic pancreatitis: A life experience; in Beger HG, Büchler M, Ditschuneit H, Malfertheimer P (eds): Berlin, Springer, 1990, pp 47–62.

6 Prinz RA, Greenlee HB: Pancreatic duct drainage in 100 patients with chronic pancreatitis. Ann Surg 1981;313–318.

7 Bradley EL III: Pseudocysts in chronic pancreatitis: Development in clinical implications; in Beger HG, Büchler M, Malfertheimer P (eds): Chronic Pancreatitis. Berlin, Springer, 1990, pp 260–268.

8 Sarner M, Cotton PB: Classification of pancreatitis. Gut 1984;25:756–759.

9 Singer MV, Gyr K: Revised classification of pancreatitis. Gastroenterology 1985;89:683–690.

10 Morel P, Rohner A: Surgery for chronic pancreatitis. Surgery 1987; 101:130–134.

11 Williamson RCN, Cooper MJ: Resection in chronic pancreatitis. Br J Surg 1987;74:807–812.
12 Stone WM, Nagorney DM: Chronic pancreatitis. Results of Whipple's resection and total pancreatectomy. Arch Surg 1988;123:815–819.
13 Traverso LW, Longmire WP: Preservation of the pylorus during pancraticoduodenectomy. Surg Gynecol Obstet 1978;146:959–962.
14 Beger HG, Witte C, Krautzberger W, Bittner R: Erfahrung mit einer das Duodenum erhaltenden Pancreaskopfresection bei chronischer Pankreatitis. Chirurg 1980;51:303–308.
15 Guicherit OR, Gooszen HG, Van der Burg MPM, Lamers CBHW. Postprandial release of cholecystokinin after duodenum-preserving total pancreatectomy is independent of intraluminal pancreatic protease activity in dogs. Digestion 1990;47:226–231.
16 Inoue K, Tobe T, Suzuki T, Hosotani R, Kogire M, Fuchigami A, Miyaskita T, Tsuda K, Seino Y: Plasma cholecystokinin and pancreatic polypeptide response after radical pancreatectomy with Billroth I and Billroth II type of reconstruction. Ann Surg 1987;206:148–154.
17 Partington PF, Rochelle RE: Modified Puestow procedure for retrograde drainage of the pancreatic duct. Ann Surg 1960;152:1037–1043.
18 Linethan IP, Lambert MA, Brown DC, Kurtz AB, Cotton PB, Russell RCG: Total pancreatectomy for chronic pancreatitis. Gut 1988;29: 358–365.
19 Zirngibl H, Gall FP: Results of Whipple procedure in combination with pancreatic duct occlusion; in Berger HG, Büchler M, Ditschuneit H, Malfertheimer P (eds): Berlin, Springer, 1990, pp 481–489.
20 Rossi RL, Soeldner JS, Braasch JW, Heiss FW, Shea JA, Nugent FW, Watkins E, Silvermann ML, Bolton J: Segmental pancreatic autotransplantation with ductal occlusion for chronic pancreatitis. Ann Surg 1986;203:626–636.
21 Najarian JS, Sutherland DER, Baumgartner D, Burke B, Rynasiewicz JJ, Matas AJ, Goetz FC: Total or near total pancreatectomy and islet autotransplantation for treatment of chronic pancreatitis. Ann Surg 1980;192:526–542.

Dig Dis 1992;10:354–362

M. Büchler
W. Uhl
H.G. Beger

Department of General Surgery
University of Ulm, FRG

Acute Pancreatitis: When and How to Operate

Key Words
Acute pancreatitis
Surgical management
Indications
Necrosectomy and lavage therapy

Abstract
Patients with proved necrotizing pancreatitis should be treated in an intensive care unit. Surgical management of necrotizing pancreatitis is indicated if an acute abdomen or persistent or increasing signs of organ complications develop, such as pulmonary or renal insufficiency, cardiocirculatory dysfunction or metabolic disorders, and these do not respond to maximum intensive care treatment over at least 72 h. Besides these so-called non-responders to ICU treatment, operative management is clearly indicated in patients who develop signs of sepsis on the basis of a bacteriologically positive fine-needle aspiration of pancreatic necroses. In patients with minor necroses without any bacterial contamination and without extensive retroperitoneal fatty tissue necroses intensive care therapy can be successful without the necessity of a surgical intervention. The gold standard of surgical management of necrotizing pancreatitis is careful removal of necrotic tissue, drainage of bacterially infected area, elimination of the pancreatogenic ascites in order to prevent systemic spread of vasoactive and toxic substances and interruption of the inflammatory process. For the treatment of pancreatic necrosis we strongly support surgical debridement (necrosectomy), supplemented by postoperative closed continuous lavage of the lesser sac and the adjacent necrotic cavities. In 152 patients suffering from severe necrotizing pancreatitis the hospital mortality was 12.5% (19/152) by this surgical approach.

Markus Büchler, MD
Department of General Surgery
University of Ulm, Steinhövelstrasse 9
D-W-7900 Ulm (FRG)

© 1992
S. Karger AG, Basel
0257–2753/92/
0106–0354$2.75/0

Clinical management of acute pancreatitis is based on the observation that most patients have a mild, self-limiting disease [1–3]. However, there are appreciable uncertainties with regard to the therapeutic schedule, since a specific and effective pharmacotherapy is not available, and as the effectiveness of a surgical therapy of necrotizing pancreatitis has not been substantiated by controlled prospective clinical data up to now. Undoubtedly, in patients with acute pancreatitis and local septic complications following a bacterial contamination of necrotic material surgical therapy could be proved superior to the conservative treatment protocol [4–6].

Goals of surgical management of necrotizing pancreatitis are: removal of necrotic peri- and intrapancreatic tissue, emptying of pancreatogenic ascites in the peritoneal cavity and the lesser sac, blocking of the inflammatory and necrotizing process, in order to prevent systemic release of vasoactive and toxic substances. A further very important step in the operative therapy is the preservation of vital intact pancreatic tissue. This is based on the experience that from a macromorphological point of view the necrotizing process is often mainly represented by fatty tissue necrosis in and around the vital exocrine and endocrine pancreatic parenchyma [7, 8].

In the past, a variety of surgical treatment modalities have been propagated (table 1) including pancreatic resection [9–11], peritoneal dialysis [13, 14], multiple tube drainage [15], surgical debridement and suction drainage [5, 16], necrosectomy with postoperative continuous local lavage of necrotic cavities [17], various forms of open packing [18–21], and nonoperative drainage using percutaneous techniques [22–24]. The results of an operative therapy for necrotizing pancreatitis depend not only on the surgical technique used, but also on the patient collective, the severity of concomitant morbidity factors, timing of surgical intervention, extent of the necrotizing process and, most important, on the bacterial contamination of necroses [6, 25].

Table 1. Necrotizing pancreatitis: surgical management protocols

Pancreatic resection (Watts, 1963; Edelmann, 1974)
Peritoneal dialysis (Wall, 1965; Ranson, 1978; Mayer, 1985)
Triple-tube drainage (Lawson, 1970)
Necrosectomy/debridement + sump drainage (Watermann, 1968; Warshaw, 1986)
Open abdomen, open packing (Bolooki, 1968; Davidon, 1986)
Necrosectomy + closed lesser sac lavage (Beger, 1982)
Nonoperative drainage (Gerzof, 1981; van Sonnenberg, 1989)

Indication to Surgical Management

The development of pancreatic and/or extrapancreatic necrosis is the critical feature determining the prognosis of acute pancreatitis. For the early assessment of the severity of acute pancreatitis C-reactive protein, PMN-elastase and phospholipase A2 catalytic activity have been shown to have high accuracy rates for the detection of pancreatic necroses [26, 27]. Therefore, CT scanning [28] can be restricted today to those cases with high values of these necrosis indicating parameters, in dealing with special questions, such as the evaluation of the intra- and extrapancreatic extent of necroses.

There is no question that patients with proved severe necrotizing pancreatitis should be treated in an intensive care unit, as the early phase of the disease is characterized by organ complications such as shock, and lung

Table 2. ICU treatment of acute pancreatitis (i.v. catheter, urine catheter, gastric tube)

1	Pulmonary insufficiency	$paO_2 < 70$ mm Hg $paO_2 < 60$ mm Hg under oxygen	→ →	oxygen supply mechanical ventilation
2	Renal insufficiency	serum creatinine > 120 µmol/l urine volume < 30 ml/h	→	dopamine (low dose) + diuretics
		BUN > 30 mmol/l or serum creatinine > 400 µmol/l	→	hemofiltration hemodialysis
3	Cardiocirculatory dysfunction/shock	central venous pressure ↓ mean arterial pressure < 70 mm Hg systolic blood pressure < 90 mm Hg ≥ 10 min	→ → →	volume replacement dopamine (high dose) Swan-Ganz catheter norepinephrine
4	Metabolic disorders	hyperglycemia > 11.1 mmol/l disseminated intravascular coagulation (DIC)	→ →	insulin fresh frozen plasma
5	Sepsis	rectal temperature > 38.5 °C leukocytes < 4,000/> 12,000/mm^3 platelets < 150,000/mm^3, metabolic acidosis > –4 mmol/l	→	antibiotics surgical intervention
	Fine needle aspiration	→ infected necrosis	→	surgery
	Biliary pancreatitis (bilirubin ↑, ASAT ↑, alkaline phosphatase ↑)	endoscopic retrograde cholangiography	→	papillotomy for impacted stones

and kidney failure caused by the release of vasoactive and toxic substances [29]. A certain percentage of patients with necrotizing pancreatitis and organ complications can be successfully treated with intensive care measures and an operation can be avoided [30]. Intensive care measures imply specific therapy forms of pulmonary, renal and cardiocirculatory dysfunctions (table 2).

From a clinical point of view, surgical management is indicated in patients with necrotizing pancreatitis who develop signs of a surgical acute abdomen and septic complications caused by a bacterial contamination of necroses, primarily by gram-negative germs from the intestinal flora such as *Escherichia coli, Pseudomonas, Streptococcus fecalis,* etc.

Table 3. Necrotizing pancreatitis: indications to surgical management

Clinical criteria
1 Surgical acute abdomen
2 Sepsis syndrome
3 Shock syndrome
4 Non-response to ICU treatment (> 3 days), persisting or increasing local or systemic complications, pulmonary insufficiency, renal failure, cardiocirculatory insufficiency

Morphological + bacteriological data
Infected necroses
Extended pancreatic necroses (> 50%)
Extended intrapancreatic + retroperitoneal necroses
Stenosis of CBD, duodenum, large bowel

CBD = Common bile duct.

Table 4. Indications for surgical management of patients with proven necrotizing pancreatitis in 152 prospectively treated patients[1]

	Patients	Frequency, %
Acute surgical abdomen	12	8.0
Sepsis	67	43.0
Cardiocirculatory shock	2	1.3
MOF syndrome (despite ICU treatment ≥ 3 days)	75	48.0
Pulmonary insufficiency	86	55.0
Renal failure	12	8.0
Metabolic insufficiency	7	5.0
Persisting acute upper abdominal mass (despite ICU treatment ≥ 8 days)	49	31.0
Increase of the extent of necrosis[2]	79	51.0

[1] 5/1982–12/1990 Department of General Surgery, University of Ulm, Germany.
[2] Contrast-enhanced CT examinations.

The overall contamination rate of the necrotic material amounts to approximately 40% in the first week of the disease [6]. Persisting organ failure such as pulmonary and/or renal insufficiency, and severe gastrointestinal bleeding or metabolic disorders are indications for surgical therapy, if these complications worsen over a period of at least 3–5 days of maximum intensive care treatment. Patients who develop an upper abdominal mass with abdominal pain (despite analgesic therapy) after the second week of proved necrotizing pancreatitis, or who suffer from an increasing leukocytosis at subfebrile temperatures, and patients with increasing ileus symptoms are also candidates for surgical therapy (table 3). The assessment of non-response of the local and systemic organ complications to conservative therapy is a very important interdisciplinary step and the basis of the decision for surgery.

According to morphological criteria found by contrast-enhanced CT scanning [28] for the evaluation of intra- and extrapancreatic necroses, by fine-needle aspiration (guided by imaging procedures) [31], patients with proved infected necroses, extended pancreatic parenchymal necrosis (involving more than 50% of the gland) with or without extrapancreatic fatty tissue necroses, and with local complications such as stenosis of the common bile duct, duodenum or colon, are also candidates for surgical intervention. Patients with focal or minor necroses present a moderate clinical picture, and therefore will respond to conservative therapy [30].

Between 5/1982 and 12/1990, we observed 152 patients with necrotizing pancreatitis. An acute abdomen developed in about 8%, sepsis in about 43%, 2% had a shock syndrome, and 48% had to be operated on for systemic organ complications which had not responded to intensive care therapy. In 31% of patients persisting acute upper abdominal mass despite ICU treatment over 8 days was considered an indicator for surgical intervention. Additionally, in 51% of patients an enlargement of the necrotizing process during intensive care therapy was found (table 4).

Timing of Surgery

The operative therapy of necrotizing pancreatitis is based on an exhaustive application of conservative intensive care measures. The timing of surgical intervention in severe acute pancreatitis is still under discussion today. The intervention can be performed 'early', that is in the acute phase, if complications arise which make an early operation absolutely necessary [32, 33] or if the diagnosis is still uncertain [34], but the intervention can also be delayed [24]. The rationale for the concept of delaying surgical therapy is to wait until demarcation of the necroses has occurred. However, the problem is that the demarcation process cannot be evaluated objectively. Furthermore, there are no sufficiently objective data about the response to conservative therapy and the efficiency of maximum intensive care treatment protocols (e.g. longterm artificial respiration or hemofiltration); however, a minimum period of intensive care therapy should be observed. In the Ulm hospital, surgery was carried out on the 9th day on average (range 1–64 days) after the onset of acute abdominal symptoms, and on the fifth day (on average) of ICU treatment (range 0–56 days). Early operative intervention in the first week of the disease is only indicated in the small group of patients with fulminant necrotizing pancreatitis (subtotal to total necrosis of the pancreatic gland) and in proved early bacterial contamination of the necroses.

Techniques of Surgical Treatment

Surgical treatment of necrotizing pancreatitis centers on the removal of the necrosis and the continuous evacuation of pancreatic fluids, which may contain bacterial and biologically active compounds. Thus, peritoneal dialysis [13, 14] alone cannot be considered as an adequate therapy for acute pancreatitis, as has been demonstrated by Mayer et al. [14]. In this study, hospital mortality was the same in the control group and in the group treated with peritoneal dialysis (27 and 28%, respectively). According to current clinical studies, a significant reduction of organ complications and the mortality rate cannot be achieved nor is it to be expected, as the effects of peritoneal lavage are restricted to the abdominal cavity and have no influence on the persisting necrotizing process in the retroperitoneal spaces. This therapeutic approach does not provide for an evacuation of necrotic or bacterially infected tissue.

The exclusive operative implantation of several thick drainage tubes into the omental bursa, combined with a bile duct drainage (cholecystectomy plus T drainage), gastrostomy and jejunostomy is only partly successful, as necrosectomy is missing. This treatment form, known as the so-called 'triple tube drainage' [15] and mostly applied in American clinics from 1970 onwards, aims at the drainage of ascitic fluid from the lesser sac and the inhibition of the exocrine pancreatic secretion. Application of this surgical procedure has shown, however, that it does not lead to a substantial reduction of morbidity and mortality. As necroses and bacterially infected intra- and retropancreatic inflammatory process are not removed, it is not surprising that pancreatic abscesses grow up with a frequency of up to 40% after application of this 'triple tube drainage' [35].

Surgical treatment of necrotizing pancreatitis with the classical resection techniques, hemipancreatectomy, partial or total pancreaticoduodenectomy, aims at the total removal of the diseased pancreatic tissue or the whole organ [9–11]. Partial or total pancreaticoduodenectomy also requires the removal of otherwise healthy organs (duodenum, parts of the stomach, extrapancreatic ducts) and this

Table 5. Results of surgical debridement/necrosectomy in necrotizing pancreatitis/pancreatic abscess

Study	Patients	Hospital mortality		Hospitalization days	Postop. complications[1], %	Reoperation, %	Additional surgical technique
		n	%				
Becker, 1982	62	25	40		80	31	drainage
Warshaw, 1985	45	11 (1/19)	24 (5)	49	84	27	multiple suction drainage
Bradley, 1987	28	3	11	46	4–36	100	open packing

1 Pancreatic fistula, enteric fistula, gastric obstruction, incisional hernia, retroperitoneal hemorrhage.

imposes additional stress on the severely ill patient. Furthermore, surgeons must be aware that in quite a number of cases with necrotizing pancreatitis only the external parts of the pancreas are necrotic, the pancreatic parenchyma around the pancreatic duct being intact. This type, known as superficial necrotizing pancreatitis, can easily be mistaken by the surgeon as a total necrosis of the gland and lead to the wrong kind of treatment [7], if he does not know the overall morphology, which might be seen from a contrast-enhanced CT scan of the pancreas. Except for the very rare cases of total pancreatic necrosis, pancreatic resection involves the risk of overtreatment and increases late morbidity and mortality mainly caused by insufficiency.

As the exclusive lavage or drainage of the retroperitoneum is not able to bring down the high morbidity and mortality rate in necrotizing pancreatitis, other surgical principles, combined with debridement of necroses, were introduced in the past. In the Mayo series, published by Becker et al. [36] in 1982, the hospital mortality of patients with pancreatic abscess was 40%, and the reoperation rate 31% (table 5). The authors were dissatisfied with these results, feeling that surgical necrosectomy with drainage alone was insufficient for a significant reduction of mortality. Therefore, additional treatment protocols following surgical debridement were developed. These surgical modalities comprise the application of open packing with multiple redressing, multiple sump drainage with lavage or planned frequent reoperations with or without a zipper [11, 18–21]. Multiple redressings and frequent reoperations remove the necrosis and are carried out in combination with intraoperative lavage. The Boston series, reported by Warshaw and Jin [5], showed a significant decrease in hospital mortality of patients with necrotizing pancreatitis or pancreatic abscesses. The overall hospital mortality in the Boston series was 24%; in a later period only 1 of 19 patients died. In Atlanta, the open packing technique is applied exclusively [21]. Multiple redressings, however, entail many reoperations, a prolonged intensive-care phase, and an enormous additional stress for the patient. Multiple reoperations are also the cause of an increased occurrence of intestinal fistulae, stomach outlet stenoses, mechanical ileus, incisional herniae, and complications with local severe bleeding.

More recently, interventional techniques for the nonoperative management of necrotizing pancreatitis were introduced. Good results were reported with big drainage tubes, which were placed percutaneously in the ne-

Table 6. Necrotizing pancreatitis (NP): results of necrosectomy + continuous local lavage; prospective clinical trial 5/1982–12/1990 (152 patients)

Preoperatively	Severity of NP	3.6 Ranson points (median)
	Infected necrosis	43%
Postoperatively	Hospitalisation	66 days (median among survivors)
	Lavage duration	39 days (median)
	Lavage fluid	8 liters/24 h (median)
	Reoperation	30%
	Hospital mortality	12.5% (19/152)
	Infected necrosis	16.4% (11/67)
	Sterile necrosis	9.4% (8/85)

crotic areas [22, 23], using imaging procedures and avoiding surgical intervention completely. So far the experience with this new treatment protocol is limited, however, and obviously this method cannot guarantee the complete removal of necrotic areas. Every second patient in the van Sonnenberg et al. [23] series had to be operated after drainage, since the removal of necrotic tissue and the bacterially contaminated necroses was not efficient enough.

Ulm Protocol of Surgical Management

For the treatment of pancreatic necroses we strongly advocate surgical debridement, necrosectomy, supplemented by intraoperative and postoperative closed continuous local lavage of the lesser sac of the necrotic cavities involved [4, 14, 17]. This provides an atraumatic and continuous evacuation of devitalized necrotic tissue as well as removal of bacterially contaminated dead tissue and biologically active substances from the ongoing necrotizing process after necrosectomy. In the meantime, this procedure has been very successfully introduced into our clinical routine.

Necrosectomy and Lavage Therapy

After opening of the abdominal cavity, using an upper abdominal midline incision in most patients, the gastrocolic and duodenocolic ligaments are divided, and the pancreas is exposed. The extent of necrosis in the head, body and tail of the gland can easily be assessed and measured. Debridement of necrosectomy, either digital or by the careful use of instruments, permits the exclusive elimination of all demarcated devitalized tissue, preserving the vital pancreatic parenchymal tissue. After surgical debridement, a thorough hemostasis with transfixion stitches, using monofilament suture material, is mandatory. It has become increasingly clear that it is not necessary to remove every gram of devitalized tissue, because any tissue being or becoming necrotic is rinsed out by the lavage fluid. After the surgical debridement and suturing of bleeding vessels, an extensive intraoperative lavage is performed using 3–6 liters of normal saline, in order to clear the surface of the pancreatic and peripancreatic tissues. For the postoperative closed continuous local lavage (the necrotizing process is of course still going on) two or more large (28–34 Fr) double-lumen silicon rubber tubes are inserted, so that a regionally restricted lavage is effected at least. The gastrocolic and duodenocolic ligaments are sutured to create a closed retroperitoneal lesser sac compartment for the postoperative continuous lavage. In the first postoperative days, the amount of lavage fluid is 24 liters per tube, a fast reduction taking place during the following days, depending on the clinical course and the appearance of the outflowing liquid. For the lavage a slightly hyperosmotic fluid is used, mostly the normal CAPD solution. Lavage can be stopped as soon as there are no more signs of acute pancreatitis and after the necrotic cavities have been completely cleansed. This is confirmed by the measurement of pancreatic enzyme levels in the return fluid, assessing the sterility of the fluid, and evaluating the amount of recovered devitalized tissue. Finally, the drainage tubes are removed successively.

Up to now 152 patients with necrotizing pancreatitis have been treated with this protocol; the data resulting from this technique are given in table 6. The patients had a severe type of acute pancreatitis with 3.6 Ranson points (median value) and an infection rate of 43%. The postoperative lavage duration was 39 days, and the amount of lavage fluid was 8 liters per day in median. In the postoperative period after necrosectomy and during closed local lavage treatment systemic organ complications were rare and occurred mainly in connection with local complications. 46 patients (30%) had to be reoperated, mostly for an abscess or an ongoing necrotizing process forming in the area of the original necrotic cavity. In this patient population with the severe type of necrotizing pancreatitis hospital mortality was 12.5% (19/152). Death was mostly related to both the extent of necrosis and the presence of bacterial infection of the necroses. The mortality rate of patients with infected necroses was aproximately twice as high as that of patients with sterile pancreatic necroses (16.4 vs. 9.4%).

References

1 Warshaw AL: A guide to pancreatitis. Compreh Ther 1980;6:49–55.
2 Beger HG, Büchler M: Decision-making in surgical treatment of acute pancreatitis: Operative or conservative management of necrotizing pancreatitis? Theor Surg 1986;1: 61–68.
3 Büchler M: Objectification of the severity of acute pancreatitis. Hepatogastroenterology 1991;38:101–108.
4 Beger HG, Krautzberger W, Bittner R, Block S, Büchler M: Results of surgical treatment of necrotizing pancreatitis. World J Surg 1985;90: 972–979.
5 Warshaw AL, Jin G: Improved survival in 45 patients with pancreatic abscess. Ann Surg 1985;202:408–417.
6 Beger HG, Krautzberger W, Bittner R, Büchler M, Block S: Bacterial contamination of pancreatic necrosis. A prospective clinical study. Gastroenterology 1986;91:433–438.
7 Leger L, Chiche B, Ghouti A, Lovel A: Pancréatites aiguës nécrose capsulaire superficielle et atteinte parenchymateuse. J Chir (Paris) 1978; 115:65–70.
8 Becker V: Pathological anatomy and pathogenesis of acute pancreatitis. World J Surg 1981;5:303–313.
9 Edelmann G, Boutelier Ph: Le traitement des pancréatites aiguës nécrosantes par l'ablation chirurgicale précoce des portions nécrosées. Chirurgie 1974;100:155–167.
10 Alexandre JH, Guerreri MT: Role of total pancreatectomy in the treatment of necrotizing pancreatitis. World J Surg 1981;5:369–377.
11 Hollender LF, Meyer C, Marrie A, da Costa SE, Castellanos JG: Role of surgery in the management of acute pancreatitis. World J Surg 1981;5: 361–368.
12 Wall AJ: Peritoneal dialysis in the treatment of severe acute pancreatitis. Med J Aust 1965;ii:281–287.
13 Lasson A, Balldin G, Genell S, Ohlsson K: Peritoneal lavage in severe acute pancreatitis. Acta Chir Scand 1984;150:479–484.
14 Mayer AD, McMahon MJ, Corfield AP, Cooper MJ, Williamson RCN, Chir M: Controlled clinical trial of peritoneal lavage for the treatment of severe acute pancreatitis. N Engl J Med 1985;312:399–404.
15 McCarthy MC, Dickermann RM: Surgical management of severe acute pancreatitis. Arch Surg 1982; 117:476–480.

16 Watermann NG, Walsky RS, Kasdan ML: The treatment of acute hemorrhagic pancreatitis by sump drainage. Surg Gynecol Obstet 1968;126:963–974.
17 Beger HG, Büchler M, Bittner R, Block S, Nevalainen T, Roscher R: Necrosectomy and postoperative local lavage in necrotizing pancreatitis. Br J Surg 1988;75:207–221.
18 Knol JA, Eckhauser FE, Strodel WE: Surgical treatment of necrotizing pancreatitis by marsupialization. Am Surg 1984;50:324–328.
19 Stone HH, Strom PR, Mullins RJ: Pancreatic abscess management by subtotal resection and packing. World J Surg 1984;8:340–345.
20 Wertheimer MD, Norris CS: Surgical management of necrotizing pancreatitis. Arch Surg 1986;121:484–487.
21 Bradley EL III: Management of infected pancreatic necrosis by open drainage. Ann Surg 1987;206:542–550.
22 Gerzof SG, Robbins AJ, Johnson WC, Birkett DH, Nabseth DC: Percutanous catheter drainage of abdominal abscess: A five-year experience. N Engl J Med 1981;305:653–657.
23 van Sonnenberg E, Wing VW, Casola G, Nakamoto SK, Mueller PR, Ferrucci JT, Halasz NA, Simeone JF: Temporizing effect of percutaneous drainage of complicated abscesses in critically ill patients. AJR 1984;142:821–826.
24 Larvin M, Chlamers AG, Robinson PJ, McMahon MJ: Debridement and closed cavity irrigation for the treatment of pancreatic necrosis. Br J Surg 1989;76:465–471.
25 Büchler M, Malfertheimer P, Friess H, Bittner R, Vanek E, Schlegel P, Beger HG: The penetration of antibiotics into human pancreas. Infection 1989;17:20–25.
26 Büchler M, Malfertheimer P, Schoetensack C, Uhl W, Beger HG: Sensitivity of antiproteases, complement factors and C-reactive protein in detecting pancreatic necrosis. Results of a prospective clinical study. Int J Pancreatol 1986;1:227–235.
27 Büchler M, Malfertheimer P, Schädlich H, Nevalainen TJ, Friess H, Beger HG: Role of phospholipase A2 in human acute pancreatitis. Gastroenterology 1989;97:1521–1526.
28 Block S, Maier W, Clausen C, Bittner R, Büchler M, Malfertheimer P, Beger HG: Identification of pancreas necrosis in severe acute pancreatitis. Gut 1986;27:1035–1042.
29 Beger HG, Bittner R, Büchler M, Hess M, Schmitz JE: Hemodynamic data pattern in patients with acute pancreatitis. Gastroenterology 1986;90:74–79.
30 Büchler M, Malfertheimer P, Uhl W, Beger HG: Conservative treatment of necrotizing pancreatitis in patients with minor pancreatic necrosis. Pancreas 1988;3:592.
31 Gerzof SG, Banks PA, Robbins AH: Role of guided percutaneous aspiration in early diagnosis of pancreatic sepsis. Dig Dis Sci 1984;29:950.
32 Kivilaakso E, Fräki O, Nikki P, Lempinen M: Resection of the pancreas for acute fulminant pancreatitis. Surg Gynecol Obstet 1981;152: 493–498.
33 Poston GJ, Williamson RCN: Surgical management of acute pancreatitis. Br J Surg 1990;77:5–12.
34 Ranson JHC, Rifkind KM, Roses DF, Fink SD, Eng K, Spencer FC: Prognostic signs and the role of operative management in acute pancreatitis. Surg Gynecol Obstet 1974; 139:69–81.
35 Warshaw AL: Inflammatory masses following acute pancreatitis. Surg Clin North Am 1974;54:620–637.
36 Becker JM, Pamberton JH, DiMagno EP, Jestrup DM: Prognostic factors in pancreatic abscess. Surgery 1984;96:455–460.

Author Index

Volume 10, Supplement 1 has its own Author Index

Subject Index

Volume 10, Supplement 1 has its own Subject Index

Vol. 10, 1992

Digestive Diseases

Current Concepts in Research and Practice
Formerly 'Survey of Digestive Diseases'

Editors-in-Chief

T.S.N. Chen, East Orange, N.J.
R.P. MacDermott, Philadelphia, Pa.

Editorial Board

Infectious Disease
E.C. Boedeker, Washington, D.C.

Radiology
P.S. Chen, Worcester, Mass.

Endoscopy
D. Fleischer, Washington, D.C.

Liver
P. Ferenci, Wien
T. Kiernan, Augusta, Ga.
K. Okuda, Chiba

Pharmacology
R.G. Knodell, Baltimore, Md.
C. Scarpignato, Parma

Bile
U.A. Marbet, Basel

Immunology
S. Kakumu, Nagoya

Esophagus and Stomach
S.K. Lam, Hong Kong
D.A. Peura, Washington, D.C.
R.K.H. Wong, Washington, D.C.

Colon
P. Rozen, Tel-Aviv

Preventive Medicine
C.H. Tamburro, Louisville, Ky.

Oncology
M. Tempero, Omaha, Nebr.

Pediatric Gastroenterology
J.A. Vanderhoof, Omaha, Nebr.

Surgery
L.F. Rikkers, Omaha, Nebr.
J.S. Thompson, Omaha, Nebr.

KARGER

S. Karger
Medical and Scientific Publishers
Basel · Freiburg · Paris · London
New York · New Delhi · Bangkok
Singapore · Tokyo · Sydney

Drug Dosage
The authors and the publisher have exerted every effort to ensure that drug selection and dosage set forth in this text are in accord with current recommendations and practice at the time of publication. However, in view of ongoing research, changes in government regulations, and the constant flow of information relating to drug therapy and drug reactions, the reader is urged to check the package insert for each drug for any change in indications and dosage and for added warnings and precautions. This is particularly important when the recommended agent is a new and/or infrequently employed drug.

All rights reserved.
No part of this publication may be translated into other languages, reproduced or utilized in any form or by any means, electronic or mechanical, including photocopying, recording, microcopying, or by any information storage and retrieval system, without permission in writing from the publisher or, in the case of photocopying, direct payment of a specified fee to the Copyright Clearance Center (see 'Information for Readers and Subscribers').

© Copyright 1992 by S. Karger AG,
P.O. Box, CH–4009 Basel (Switzerland)
Printed in Switzerland on acid-free paper by
Thür AG Offsetdruck, Pratteln

Contents Vol. 10, 1992

No. 4

No. 5

No. 6

Controversies about Inflammatory Diseases of the Pancreas

Suppl. 1

KLINIKARZT

«... ein didaktisch gelungener, methodisch und inhaltlich aktueller, dabei klassischer Leitfaden durch die symptomorientierte Diagnostik der inneren Medizin ...»

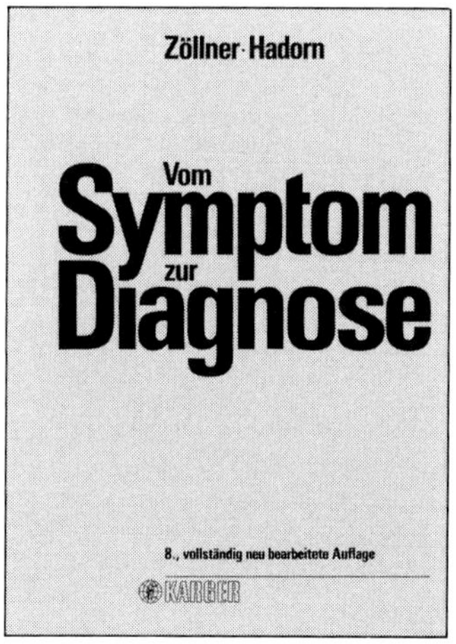

Im Unterschied zu den klassischen Lehrbüchern der Medizin sind die einzelnen Kapitel dieses Buches symptomorientiert und damit praxisnah aufgebaut. Besonderer Wert wird auf die Anamnese und die klinische Beobachtung gelegt; didaktisch vorzügliche Tabellen und Abbildungen helfen, die Entscheidungsfindung zu beschleunigen. Die Differentialdiagnose der häufigen und lebensbedrohenden Krankheiten steht stets im Vordergrund. Ein reichhaltiges Sachregister erleichtert das rasche Auffinden der Symptome und Krankheitsbilder.
«Vom Symptom zur Diagnose» enthält in knapper Form alle Informationen, die der Praktiker für seine Differentialdiagnose benötigt. Der nichtinternistische Facharzt findet wichtige diagnostische Hinweise für Fälle, welche die Grenzen seines Fachgebietes überschreiten. Dem Studenten dient das Lehrbuch zur Integration und damit der praktischen Anwendung seines klinischen Wissens.

Vom Symptom zur Diagnose
Herausgeber: N. Zöllner, München; W. Hadorn, Bern
8., vollständig neubearbeitete Auflage
X + 682 S., 249 Schwarzweiss- und 56 Farbabb., 317 Tab., gebunden, 1986
SFr. 124.– / DM 148.– / £ 54.00 / US$ 99.25
Preisänderungen vorbehalten
DM-Preise nur für BRD, £-Preise nur für GB, US $-Preise nur für USA
ISBN 3-8055-4030-2

KARGER

KI 92776

Issues in Biomedicine. Monographs in Interdisciplinary Topics (ISSN 1010–8408), **Vol. 15**
Series Editors: H. Stolte, Hannover; R.K.H. Kinne, Dortmund; P.H. Bach, London

Biology and Medicine into the 21st Century

Editors:
M.A. Hardy
R.K.H. Kinne

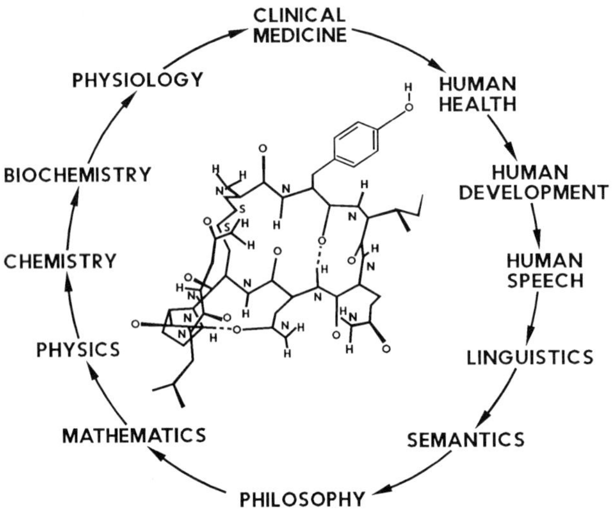

Special price for readers of Karger journals: SFr. 123.– / DM 147.– / £ 53.50 / US$ 98.00

This unique publication combines thorough reviews of progress in key areas of biomedical research with provocative reflections on the intellectual, social and ethical problems biology and medicine will be facing in the foreseeable future. The contributions range from investigations to elucidate the molecular mechanisms underlying cellular functions to consideration of the complex interactions between science and society. Examples of such interplay illustrate the impact of biomedical research on society and how the boundary conditions set by the latter determine the success of the former. Establishing a fascinating dialogue between eminent experts in biology, medicine and health care, including several Nobel laureates, this book offers rewarding reading to clinicians, basic scientists, sociologists, and professionals in medical education and health care management.

Fields of Interest

Natural Sciences for Physicians; Molecular Biology, Biochemistry, Physiology; Biology for Physicians, Biophysics, Cell Biology, Neurology, Oncology, Radiology

Contents

Kinne, R.K.H.; Eggena, P.: Basic Sciences and Medicine in the Career of Irving L. Schwartz
Hechter, O.: Reflections on the Future of Biomedical Science
Huberman, *B.A.:* The Collective Mind
Rasmussen, H.: Disordered Cell Communication as the Basis of Human Disease: Implications for 21st-Century Medicine
Kinne, R.K.H.: From Diversity to Similarity in Biological Transport
Kirchberger, M.A.: Phospholamban: A Molecule for the Future
Wyssbrod, H.R.; Laws, W.R.; Merrfield, R.B.: Peptide Biology: Progress and Prospects
Watson, J.D.: Reflections on Oncogenes and Antioncogenes
Baulieu, E.-E.: RU 486, an Antisteroid Molecule: Cellular Mechanism and Clinical Uses
Relman, A.S.: America's Health Care System in Transition
Yalow, R.S.: Radiation and Society
Feinstein, A.R.: Basic Clinimetric Science in 21st-Century Clinical Medicine

Issues in Biomedicine. Monographs in Interdisciplinary Topics, Vol. 15
Biology and Medicine into the 21st Century
Editors: Hardy, M.A. (New York, N.Y.); Kinne, R.K.H. (Dortmund)
VIII + 200 p., 34 fig., 5 tab., hard cover, 1991
SFr. 225.– / DM 269.– / £ 97.90 / US$ 180.00
US$ price for USA, £ price for UK only (subject to change)
ISBN 3–8055–5392–7

KARGER

KI91581